Mosby's Color Atlas and Text of

Infectious
Diseases

Commissioning Editor: Timothy Horne
Project Development: Gina Almond, Maria Stewart, Fiona Conn
Project Management: Fiona Conn, Frances Affleck
Design Direction: Judith Wright
Layout Artist: Alan Palfreyman

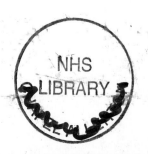

Mosby's Color Atlas and Text of

Infectious Diseases

Christopher P Conlon MA MD FRCP
Consultant Physician in Infectious Diseases
John Radcliffe Hospital, Oxford
and
Hon Senior Lecturer in Infectious Diseases
and Tropical Medicine
University of Oxford
UK

David R Snydman MD
Chief, Division of Geographic Medicine
and Infectious Disease
New England Medical Center
and
Professor of Medicine and Pathology
Tufts University School of Medicine
Boston
USA

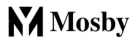 **Mosby**

EDINBURGH LONDON NEW YORK OXFORD PHILADELPHIA ST LOUIS SYDNEY TORONTO 2000

MOSBY
An imprint of Elsevier Limited

© Mosby International Limited 2002
© Elsevier Science Limited 2002
© Elsevier Limited 2004. All rights reserved.

First edition 2000
  Reprinted 2002, 2004

ISBN 0 723424349

British Library Cataloguing in Publication Data
A catalogue record for this book is available from the British Library

Library of Congress Cataloging in Publication Data
A catalog record for this book is available from the Library of Congress

Note
Medical knowledge is constantly changing. As new information becomes available, changes in treatment, procedures, equipment and the use of drugs become necessary. The author and the publishers have, as far as it is possible, taken care to ensure that the information given in this text is accurate and up to date. However, readers are strongly advised to confirm that the information, especially with regard to drug usage, complies with the latest legislation and standards of practice.

 ELSEVIER SCIENCE your source for books, journals and multimedia in the health sciences
www.elsevierhealth.com

The
publisher's
policy is to use
**paper manufactured
from sustainable forests**

Printed in China
C/03

Contents

Chapter 1   Microbes, the Host and Sepsis   1

Chapter 2   The Laboratory   9

Chapter 3   Hospital-Acquired Infections   19

Chapter 4   Principles of Epidemiology   29

Chapter 5   Cardiovascular Infection   37

Chapter 6   Infections Involving the Respiratory Tract   53

Chapter 7   Central Nervous System Infections   77

Chapter 8   Ocular Infections   89

Chapter 9   Gastrointestinal Tract and Liver, Gall Bladder and Pancreas   99

Chapter 10   Urinary and Genital Tract Infections   125

Chapter 11   Skin and Soft Tissue Infections   155

Chapter 12   Bone and Joint Infections   175

Chapter 13   The Immunocompromised Host   189

Chapter 14   Congenital and Perinatal Infections   211

Chapter 15   Tropical Infections   217

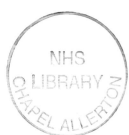

Foreword

The retained image is often critical to the diagnosis of infection. An astute clinician relies on visual clues to retrace the footprints of memories and associations with a patient's condition, some gathered from past experience and others from a book or atlas. This volume by Conlon and Snydman provides vivid photographs of common and not-so-common illnesses that all health care providers should have stencilled in their minds. Revisiting these pictures serves to reinforce this memory bank, as well as introduce some new images which could prove decisive in the diagnosis of a difficult case. While our memory may fade, the virtues of a printed record are its permanence and its availability for continuing study. The addition of the accompanying text not only reinforces the pictures, but also gives guidance in differential diagnosis and treatment.

The most rapid diagnosis of infection is achieved by a comprehensive physical examination by an experienced clinician. The traditional exercise of the art of Medicine by recognizing classic signs and symptoms of a specific infection can lead to early diagnosis and initiation of treatment before the blood sample even arrives in the laboratory. In some infections, such as meningococcaemia or lobar pneumonia, the outcome is time-sensitive, related to prompt antimicrobial treatment. In other instances, the initial choice of antibiotics is directed to specific pathogens based on visual recognition of the condition, for example, an anaerobic skin infection that requires a specific antimicrobial agent for this type of pathogen.

The transatlantic collaboration of two experienced clinicians, Christopher Conlon and David Snydman, brings together the best of the European and American traditions in management of infectious diseases. Having observed each of them on ward rounds, which is the true testing ground of any practitioner of Medicine, it is clear that they have distilled their years of bedside experience into this clear, comprehensive book, which should be a valuable source of reference in the management of infectious diseases.

Sherwood L. Gorbach, M.D.
Tufts University School of Medicine

Preface

Infectious diseases, like many medical specialities, is developing rapidly and yet is less dependent on technology than it is on careful history taking and the use of clinical skills. The continued challenges of HIV infection, the emergence of new infections and the recognition of the problems of nosocomial infection all contribute to make this an exciting branch of medicine. We hope that this book will stimulate students and young doctors to learn more about infectious processes and, perhaps, pursue some of the many questions and challenges still remaining in the field of infection. It is also possible that older general physicians will find this a useful aid in differential diagnosis. It is as true today as it was in Osler's time that much can be learned from the study of the patient at the bedside; we trust that this book will help in that learning process.

Dedication

This book is dedicated to our wives Jenny and Diane, with many thanks for putting up with us during its long gestation, and to our children: Sophie, Laura and Alex.

Acknowledgements

We are extremely grateful to the staff at Mosby for their forebearance and for their encouragement in getting us through to the final product. Thanks are also due to the staff of Oxford Medical Illustration (John Radcliffe Hospital) for all of their efforts. Finally, we acknowledge all of those who helped gather the images used and, especially our thanks go to the many patients who have allowed us to use their photographs.

Picture Acknowledgements
This book contains a large number of clinical slides, many of which have been given to us by generous friends and colleagues. We would particularly like to thank Patrick French, Peggy Frith, Fergus Gleeson, Geoff Pasvol, David Warrell and Bryan Warren. Others gratefully acknowledged are L Adelman, P Anslow, N Athansou, W Bailey, A Banning, H Barza, G Bates, S Bedri, N Beeching, M Benson, A Berendt, G Bird, J Britton, M Burch, S Burge, I Byren, C Carne, R Chapman, M Charnock, P Cooper, N Cowan, P Daoust, R Davidson, D Davies, R Davies, N Day, C Deguine, D Denning, S Eyken, K Fleming, C Garrard, B Gazzard, T Goodacre, S Gorbach, W Gray, D Hamer, P Hay, J Hayman, P Heath, R Herman, J Hopkin, I Isesley, K Ives, N Jacobus, P Jenks, M Kapembwa, S Knight, J Kurtz, A Lessing, A Lowes, S Lucas, G Luzzi, D Mabey, C MacDougall, D Mason, P Mason, P McLardy-Smith, D McGowan, A McShane, H Meissner, P Millard, N Moore, N Mortensen, R Moxon, S Nade, D Nolan, E Olesen, P Openshaw, R Pollack, P Richardson, J Roake, T Ryan, J Sanchez, G Scott, B Shepstone, C Strachan, B Sullivan, F Tally, A Thompson, J Trowell, D Waghorn, A Warin, W Weir, N White, M Wilcox, P Wordsworth.

chapter 1

Microbes, the Host and Sepsis

INFECTIOUS DISEASES – AN INTRODUCTION

The speciality of infectious diseases encompasses a wide variety of clinical areas. Some micro-organisms may cause specific infections such as hepatitis, while having little effect on the rest of the body. Other micro-organisms, such as *Staphylococcus aureus*, can sometimes cause local disease, such as impetigo, or can disseminate and affect many organ systems. The differential diagnosis of patients with suspected sepsis is broad and its elaboration requires a systematic approach (**Fig. 1.1**).

The clinical history is important in all realms of medical practice. In patients with infectious disease, aspects of the history that need to be emphasized include:
- a travel history;
- a history of exposure to environmental risks and to others with infection; and
- a history of previous serious infection (perhaps suggesting immunocompromise).

Clinical examination needs to look for foci of infection and, because signs change as infections progress, the examination should be repeated over time.

Whatever the pathological process, the management of patients with infection requires close co-operation between the clinician and the laboratories, especially the microbiology laboratory. Knowledge of the epidemiology of micro-organisms and their pathogenic mechanisms enable a better understanding of disease processes and may allow more focused investigation of the sick patient. Successful treatment relies on a good working knowledge of antimicrobial agents along with the recognition of the role of surgery and interventional radiology in obtaining appropriate microbiological specimens and removing foci of infection.

HOW DO MICRO-ORGANISMS CAUSE DISEASE?

Although a detailed account of the pathogenesis of infection is beyond the scope of this book, a brief outline of some of the mechanisms involved can be helpful.

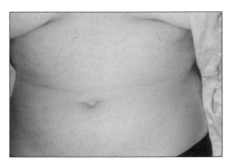

Fig. 1.1 *Many patients with systemic infections may have a skin rash, which is usually nonspecific.*

ADHERENCE

Most bacteria have to grow on some sort of surface; when they interact with humans, these organisms usually initially colonize a mucosal surface. Some streptococci are specifically adapted to colonize the oropharynx and adhere to epithelial cells in the mouth. Some strains of *Escherichia coli* produce surface antigens that allow specific adhesion to urothelial cells rather than colonic epithelium, increasing the risk of urinary tract infection. Many antigens expressed by bacteria to promote adherence are encoded by plasmids and may thus be transferable to other bacteria.

TOXINS

Numerous bacteria elaborate a variety of toxins that may either facilitate invasion by the bacteria or damage the host in some way.

Endotoxin, or lipopolysaccharide, is a constituent of the bacterial cell wall of Gram-negative organisms.

Exotoxins, on the other hand, are produced and secreted by bacteria and can have a variety of effects. For example, cholera toxin specifically affects enzymes in the small bowel mucosa that are responsible for ion and water transport, leading to profuse diarrhoea. *S. aureus* produces a variety of toxins, one of which is toxic shock syndrome toxin-1 (TSST-1). This toxin can act as a superantigen, leading to T-lymphocyte proliferation. The resulting cytokine release can lead to a myriad of clinical problems.

INVASION

Once organisms have become adherent to an epithelial surface and established colonization, they need to invade the host in order to cause disease. This may be facilitated by defects in the host but it often depends on a variety of bacterial attributes. For example, some Gram-negative bacteria have a protective cell wall that makes them relatively resistant to lysis by the host. The outer membrane proteins of these organisms may form a layer that blocks the attachment of antibody or complement so that the bacteria can evade the immune system. Gram-positive organisms, such as *Streptococcus pneumoniae*, have a thick polysaccharide capsule that is antigenically variable and often quite resistant to phagocytosis by host cells. Other organisms, such as mycobacteria, may be phagocytosed but can evade intracellular killing by remaining inside the phagosome and inhibiting fusion between the phagosome and the lysosome.

HOST DEFENCES

The human host has several layers of defence against infection, ranging from physical barriers through phagocytic cells to specialized lymphocytes.

PHYSICAL BARRIERS

The skin acts as an important barrier to infection. Keratin provides a tough and water-resistant shield against the invasion of organisms that may colonize the skin surface. In addition, specialized cells within the dermis provide immunological defences. Mucous membranes, as well as acting as physical barriers, also produce mucus as an extra defence; some, like the respiratory epithelium, are ciliated so that organisms and debris can be wafted away to the outside. The low pH of the gastric contents is a safeguard against ingested organisms and the regular and complete emptying of the urinary bladder reduces the chances of infection being established in the urinary tract.

COMPLEMENT SYSTEM

The complement system is an important component of host defences and consists of a group of highly regulated proteins and cell membrane receptors. The key elements in defence against infection are the third component (C3) and the terminal components (C5–C9). Complement can be activated by the 'classical pathway' when antigen-antibody complexes bind to and activate the first complement component (C1). C3 can be activated directly, via the 'alternative pathway', which does not depend on the presence of antibody.

The activation of complement leads to a variety of inflammatory responses, including increasing vascular permeability and neutrophil chemotaxis. Activated C3 acts as a potent opsonin when bound to micro-organisms.

There is a spectrum of inherited complement deficiencies that result in increased susceptibility to certain infections. For example, deficiency of the terminal complement components can render the person susceptible to recurrent meningococcal disease.

PHAGOCYTOSIS

The polymorphonuclear leucocyte, or neutrophil, accounts for most of the circulating white cells in the blood. Neutrophils move in an amoeboid fashion along the surface of vessels and can change shape, moving between endothelial cells and into the tissues. These phagocytes are attracted to sites of inflammation by chemotactic signals from other cells and become activated. Phagocytosis is stimulated by the binding of the Fc portion of IgG or C3 to the neutrophil membrane. The infecting organism is engulfed by a neutrophil pseudopod and a 'phagosome' is formed. Granules within the neutrophil fuse with the phagosome, releasing various microbicidal proteins, such as lysozyme. Neutrophils can also produce large quantities of hydrogen peroxide and other oxidants that act to damage bacteria. In chronic granulomatous disease, an inherited defect occurs in the polymorphs so that they are not able to undergo the respiratory burst required to generate these microbicidal products. Reductions in the number of circulating neutrophils (e.g. after cancer chemotherapy) or abnormalities in their function (e.g. in congenital adhesion defects) can lead to recurrent infection.

Monocytes and macrophages are also important phagocytes involved in host defence against infection, particularly in the tissues.

CELL-MEDIATED IMMUNITY

T lymphocytes are the mainstay of cell-mediated immunity. Antigens need to be processed by antigen-presenting cells and presented to the T-lymphocyte receptor in association with major histocompatibility complex (MHC) molecules on the cell surface. Binding to the T-lymphocyte receptor can then trigger a series of events, depending on the T lymphocyte type. The release of cytokines, such as interferon-γ and interleukin (IL)-2, by type 1 T-helper lymphocytes can help to recruit macrophages and promote phagocytosis. Cytotoxic T lymphocytes recognize and kill cells expressing foreign antigen in association with MHC Class I molecules. This is an important means of defence against viral infections. In addition, a small percentage of lymphocytes, called natural killer cells, can be activated by IL-2 and can directly kill some bacteria and virally infected cells.

HUMORAL IMMUNITY

Antibodies, in the form of immunoglobulins, form the basis of the humoral immune system. B lymphocytes differentiate into antibody-secreting plasma cells when they are stimulated by the presence of antigen. Antigen binds to B lymphocytes via cell surface immunoglobulin (acting as the B-lymphocyte receptor) and the B lymphocyte differentiates into an antibody-producing cell when stimulated by cytokines, such as IL-4 and IL-10, released from type 1 T-helper lymphocytes. Deficiencies of immunoglobulin may lead to recurrent pyogenic infections, particularly with encapsulated bacteria such as the pneumococcus.

Sites of action of antimicrobial agents

Bacterial cell wall
  B-lactams
  (penicillins, cephalosporins,
  carbapenems, monobactams)
  Glycopeptides
  Cycloserine

Fungal cytoplasmic membranes
  Amphotericin B
  Imidazoles
  Nystatin
  Terbinafine

Metabolism
  Sulphonamides
  Trimethoprim
  Isoniazid

Nucleic acid synthesis
  Quinolones
  Rifamycins
  Metronidazole
  Nitrofurantoin

Protein synthesis
  Aminoglycosides
  Tetracyclines
  Macrolides
  Clindamycin
  Fusidic acid
  Chloramphenicol
  5 Flucytosine
  Streptogramins
  Oxazolidinones

Fig. 1.2 *Classes of antibiotics and modes of action.*

ANTIBIOTICS

There are now numerous antibiotics available with which to treat bacterial infections. Knowledge of the classes of antibiotics, their mechanism of action, their likely targets and the mechanisms of antibiotic resistance are all important in the management of infectious disease. Detailed discussion is not possible here but the main antibiotic classes and their mechanisms of actions are shown in **Figure 1.2**. The distinction between bacteriostatic agents and bactericidal agents is not always important but it can be crucial in some clinical settings. Infections of the central nervous system, such as bacterial meningitis, require bactericidal antibiotics, partly because the brain is an immunologically 'privileged' site. Bactericidal agents are also required in endocarditis and osteomyelitis. Abnormalities in the host also mandate the use of bactericidal drugs (e.g. in patients with neutropenic sepsis).

SEPSIS

The term sepsis usually refers to clinical evidence of infection as well as signs of a systemic response to that infection (**Fig. 1.3**). In sepsis there is a tachycardia and increased respiratory rate, along with a fever of >38°C or an abnormal temperature response to infection (temperature <36°C). In addition, there may be a raised peripheral white cell count (>12.0×10^9/l) or the presence of immature neutrophils in the circulation. Sepsis may be caused by a variety of infectious agents that are able to breach host defences in some way so that normally sterile sites are invaded. The risk factors for sepsis are shown in **Figure 1.4**.

Sepsis and its sequelae have been defined in detail by Bone, and this has led to the concept of sepsis syndrome and septic shock (**Fig. 1.5**). In severe sepsis there is evidence of organ dysfunction, such as oliguria, confusion, hypotension, hypoxaemia, acidosis and abnormal liver function. In septic shock, hypotension persists despite adequate fluid replacement.

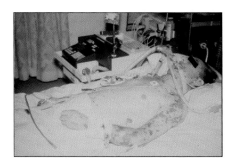

Fig. 1.3 *This patient developed shock with meningococcal septicaemia, requiring intensive care support.*

Risk factors for the development of sepsis

Extremes of age

Chronic medical condition

Indwelling device (e.g. intravenous cannula, urinary catheter)

Surgery or trauma

Hospitalization (especially in the intensive care unit)

Fig. 1.4 *Risk factors for the development of sepsis.*

Bone's criteria for sepsis

1. Body temperature >38°C or <36°C

2. Heart rate >90 beats per minute

3. Respiratory rate >20 breaths per minute
or
PCO_2 <4kPa (reflecting hyperventilation)

4. White blood cell count >12×10^9/l or <4×10^9/l
or
>10% immature polymorphs (band forms)

Fig. 1.5 *Bone's criteria for sepsis (PCO_2 = partial pressure of carbon dioxide). Adapted from Bone et al. Chest 1992;101:1644–55.*

In clinical terms, there are often rigors in association with fever. There may be evidence of increased cardiac output and warm peripheries before shock becomes established. There may be an obvious focus of infection, such as a pneumonia, but sometimes a focus is difficult to determine initially. Complications include the development of adult respiratory distress syndrome, renal failure and disseminated intravascular coagulation.

PATHOGENESIS OF SEVERE SEPSIS

Classically, septic shock is the result of the action of endotoxin released from Gram-negative bacteria. These organisms contain lipopolysaccharide, also called endotoxin, within the bacterial cell wall. When released from the bacteria (e.g. when lysed by the host immune response), lipopolysaccharide binds, via specific receptors, to macrophages and neutrophils. These cells are then stimulated to migrate and to secrete a variety of products, including cytokines. Other bacterial products can also activate the immune system. Gram-positive bacteria, such as *S. aureus* and *Streptococcus pyogenes*, produce exotoxins that have a variety of effects. Some of these exotoxins (e.g. TSST-1) can act as superantigens and bind directly to the T-lymphocyte cell receptor and the MHC Class II molecule on antigen-presenting cells, leading to extensive T-lymphocyte proliferation and cytokine release.

MEDIATORS OF SEPSIS

The activation of white cells and the immune response by infecting organisms leads to the production of a variety of chemical mediators of sepsis (**Fig. 1.6**). Cytokines, such as tumour necrosis factor-α, interleukin-1 and interferon-γ are increased in sepsis, and very high levels correlate with poorer outcomes. Arachidonic acid, a breakdown product of cell membranes, is metabolized to thromboxane and leukotrienes, which have been implicated in the pathogenesis of adult respiratory distress syndrome, as has platelet activating factor. Nitric oxide synthesis by endothelial cells can be increased by lipopolysaccharide and various cytokines. In addition, sepsis leads to the up-regulation of various adhesion molecules on endothelial cells and increases recruitment of white cells to the sites of inflammation.

In addition to the cascades of cytokines and other mediators that are set in motion by infection, there are a number of counter-regulatory events that need to occur to balance the reaction and, eventually, to curtail the inflammatory response.

PATHOPHYSIOLOGY

As a consequence of sepsis, the various mediators described above lead to organ dysfunction and, ultimately, to death of cells. An initial response to sepsis is peripheral vasodilatation, due in part to increased production of nitric oxide. The cardiac output increases as a result but this increase is insufficient to compensate for the peripheral vasodilatation, partly because some of the cytokines involved in sepsis have a direct inhibitory effect on myocardial contractility. If the heart cannot cope with demand and the peripheral vasodilatation continues, septic shock will ensue (**Fig. 1.7**).

In addition to impairing the cardiovascular system, sepsis also directly affects the lungs. Activated neutrophils migrate to and adhere to pulmonary endothelium and, with cytokines, disrupt the integrity of the endothelium. The resulting inflammation and fluid leakage lead to adult respiratory distress syndrome and thus exacerbate the hypoxia resulting from cardiovascular compromise. Local tissue hypoxia in turn leads to acidosis and may affect the coagulation system.

Mediators of sepsis	
Cytokines	Tumour necrosis factor-α Interleukin-1 Interleukin-8 Interferon-γ
Arachidonic acid metabolites	Prostaglandins Thromboxane-A$_2$ Leukotrienes
Platelet-activating factor	
Complement	
Tissue factor (in coagulation cascade)	
Nitric Oxide	

Fig. 1.6 *Mediators of sepsis.*

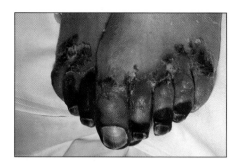

Fig. 1.7 *Peripheral gangrene secondary to septic shock.*

INVESTIGATIONS

There are no specific investigations that delineate severe sepsis. Clearly, positive cultures (e.g. of blood, cerebrospinal fluid or urine) or specific imaging may identify the infective cause. Other tests help to identify the severity of the sepsis and the degree of organ damage. The blood film may occasionally show a marked neutropenia but it usually shows a neutrophil leukocytosis and a 'left shift' in the neutrophils (i.e. more immature neutrophils are seen in the peripheral blood). Renal and hepatic function may be impaired on biochemical testing and, in particular, there may be rapid and abrupt decreases in plasma albumin. There may be evidence of disseminated intravascular coagulation, with decreased numbers of circulating platelets, impaired clotting and fragmented red cells seen on the films. Blood gases may reveal hypoxia and acidosis.

MANAGEMENT

The principles of the management of sepsis are to identify and treat the source of the sepsis while preserving tissue oxygenation. It is often not possible to define the infection clearly at the outset, so in many cases empiric, broad-spectrum antibiotic therapy is required. The choice of antimicrobial agents is guided by:
- the likely sites of infection;
- knowledge of local resistance patterns (especially in nosocomial infections);
- the extent of the patient's immunosuppression; and
- the presence of any antibiotic hypersensitivity in the patient.

In addition, surgical intervention may be required to drain abscesses or remove necrotic tissue or prosthetic material.

A key element in management is to maintain the circulation and provide respiratory support if required. Thus, early admission to an intensive care unit should be considered to ensure appropriate physiological support until more specific therapy can have an effect.

Because of the known role of inflammatory cytokines in sepsis, a variety of interventions have been tried over the years in an attempt to reduce mortality. Corticosteroids, despite having anti-inflammatory properties, have been shown not to be of benefit in septicaemia. Disappointingly, more specific therapies, such as anti-lipopolysaccharide or anti-tumour necrosis factor antibodies, have failed to have any impact on the outcome in patients with sepsis and they may even be deleterious. Many of these sorts of treatments are probably used too late in the sequence of events initiated by invasive infections. The heterogeneous nature of sepsis also means that trials of novel therapies are exceedingly difficult to conduct and interpret.

chapter 2

The Laboratory

The laboratory serves a very important function in the determination of the types of microbes that cause disease in humans. Micro-organisms are classified on the basis of:

- their Gram stain morphology;
- their colonial morphology on culture media;
- their growth characteristics;
- their biochemical reactions;
- their metabolic reactions;
- their nucleic acid composition;
- their ability to form spores; and
- serological tests, which may differentiate one species from another.

In addition, the laboratory can determine the susceptibility of the organism to antimicrobial chemotherapeutic agents in order to provide information so that the treating physician may choose the most appropriate drug.

Adequate specimens are necessary to make a microbiological diagnosis.

THE GRAM STAIN

There is probably no single procedure in clinical microbiology as important as the Gram stain. The Gram stain is used to classify organisms into one of two classes:

- Gram-positive organisms, which stain blue; and
- Gram-negative organisms, which stain red or pink.

This fundamental differentiation is central to all bacteriology.

Examples of Gram-positive and Gram-negative organisms are listed in **Figure 2.1**. The technique is outlined in **Figure 2.2**.

Gram-positive and Gram-negative Common bacteria	
Gram-Positive	**Gram-Negative**
Staphylococcus aureus	Escherichia coli
Staphylococcus epidermidis	Pseudomonas aeruginosa
Streptococcus pneumoniae	Hemophilus influenzae
Streptococci spp.	Neisseria gonorrheae
Clostridia spp.	Neisseria meningitidis
Listeria monocytogenes	Bacteroides spp.

Fig. 2.1 *Examples of Gram-positive and Gram-negative bacteria.*

Gram staining technique

1. Heat fix the material to the slide

2. Flood the slide with crystal violet and let it sit for 30 seconds

3. Wash the slide with water

4. Flood the slide with Gram's iodine and let it sit for 30 seconds

5. Wash the slide with water

6. Add alcohol-acetone to the slide while holding at an angle and allow the blue colour to wash off (1–5 seconds)

7. Flood the slide with safranin dye and let it stand for 30 seconds

8. Wash the slide with water

Fig. 2.2 *Technique for performance of the Gram stain.*

Examples of organisms with a characteristic appearance on Gram stain include *Staphylococcus aureus*, which has a distinct grape-like cluster appearance (**Fig. 2.3**), and *Streptococcus pneumoniae*, which appears classically as lancet-shaped Gram-positive diplococci (**Fig. 2.4**). Other streptococci appear as chains of Gram-positive cocci (**Fig. 2.5**). The Gram-positive rod-shaped appearance of clostridia have a distinct shape as well and have been termed 'box-car' in shape (**Fig. 2.6**).

Gram-negative organisms appear red or pink on Gram stain. Some, such as *Haemophilus influenzae*, have a coccobacillary appearance (**Fig. 2.7**) and may be very difficult to visualize owing to their light staining characteristics. Others, such as *Escherichia coli*, are more intensely staining Gram-negative rods (**Fig. 2.8**). *Neisseria meningitidis* and *Neisseria gonorrhoeae* are Gram-negative diplococci with a distinct appearance like paired coffee beans (**Fig. 2.9**).

The Gram stain is very useful because it can be applied directly to a specimen such as sputum, cerebrospinal fluid or culture plate. However, the Gram stain is still a relatively insensitive test and the specimen must contain about 100,000 organisms/ml before visualization is possible.

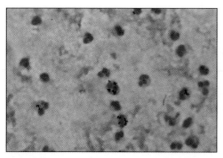

Fig. 2.3 *Gram stain of* Staphylococcus aureus.

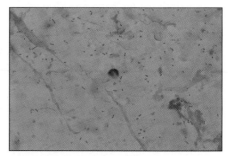

Fig. 2.4 *Gram stain of* Streptococcus pneumoniae.

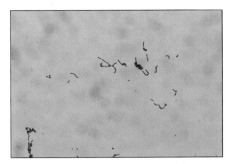

Fig. 2.5 *Gram stain of streptococci.*

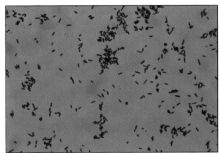

Fig. 2.6 *Gram stain of* Clostridium perfringens.

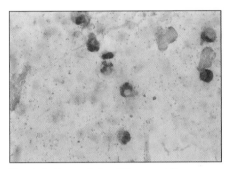

Fig. 2.7 *Gram stain of* Haemophilus influenzae.

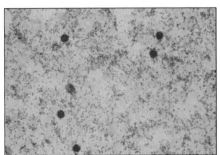

Fig. 2.8 *Gram stain of* Escherichia coli.

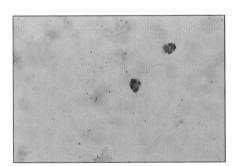

Fig. 2.9 *Gram stain of* Neisseria meningitidis.

OTHER STAINING TECHNIQUES

There are a number of other stains used in clinical microbiology. The Ziehl–Neelsen stain is used to detect mycobacteria, which possess a lipid-rich cell wall that retains the pink dye (carbol fuschia) and is not decolourized by acid-alcohol (**Fig. 2.10**). Fluorescent stains with

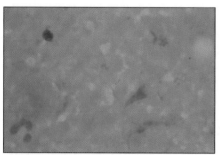

Fig. 2.10 *Ziehl-Neelsen (acid-fast) stain of* Mycobacterium tuberculosis.

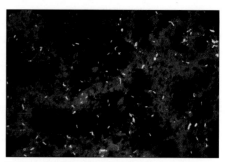

Fig. 2.11 *Auramine–rhodamine stain of* Mycobacterium tuberculosis.

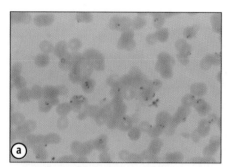

Fig. 2.12 *Thin blood films (Giemsa stain) showing (a)* Plasmodium falciparum *trophozoites (ring forms); (b)* Plasmodium vivax *late trophozoites.*

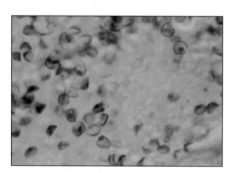

Fig. 2.13 *Gomori stain of* Pneumocystis carinii.

auramine–rhodamine can also distinguish mycobacteria (**Fig. 2.11**). These stains are more sensitive but slightly less specific than the Ziehl–Neelsen stain. Other stains of note include the Giemsa stain to detect malaria (**Fig. 2.12**) and the Gomori stain for detection of *Pneumocystis carinii* (**Fig. 2.13**).

Immunofluorescence techniques are very widely used for direct examination looking for specific pathogens. For example, direct fluorescence of the scraping of a skin lesion for varicella-zoster virus (VZV) can detect the presence of the virus by using specific antibody coupled with fluorescein dye.

CULTURE METHODS

Culture methods using agar plates are used to grow bacteria and fungi. Nonselective media using sheep blood in an agar growth medium are used for standard culturing techniques. Organisms can be classified according to their requirements for oxygen:

- those that can grow without oxygen are anaerobic organisms;
- those that require reduced oxygen and increased carbon dioxide are microaerophilic organisms; and
- those that can grow in the presence or absence of oxygen are facultative organisms.

There are selective media that are used to grow more fastidious organisms, such as *H. influenzae* (**Fig. 2.14**), *N. gonorrhoeae* or *Legionella* spp. (**Fig. 2.15**).

Selective media may be used to suppress growth of normal flora, such as that found in the stool, in order to allow the growth of pathogens such as *Salmonella* spp. (**Fig. 2.16**), *Shigella* spp. or *Campylobacter* spp. (**Fig. 2.17**). In order to provide very rapid identification of lactose-fermenting organisms, such as *E. coli*, use can be made of media that incorporate chemicals such as bile salts combined with a dye and a sugar, such as lactose, that can be fermented (**Fig. 2.18**).

Culture allows the identification and propagation of organisms, so that the bacteria can be characterized, isolates purified, and susceptibility testing performed. A major limitation in the use of culture techniques is the time it takes for organisms to be grown and the lack of sensitivity of culture when fastidious organisms may be present or when small quantities of organisms may exist at the site sampled.

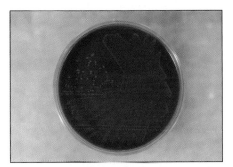

Fig. 2.14 *Chocolate agar showing growth of* **Haemophilus influenzae.**

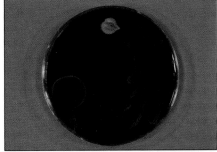

Fig. 2.15 **Legionella** *spp. growth on selective media.*

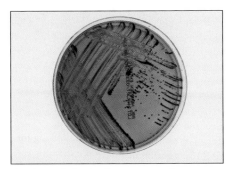

Fig. 2.16 **Salmonella** *spp. growth on* **Hektoen enteric media.**

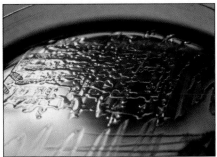

Fig. 2.17 **Campylobacter** *spp. growth on selective media.*

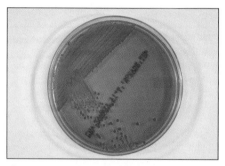

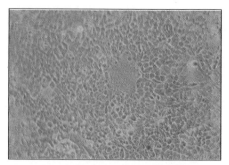

Fig. 2.18 *MacConkey plate showing lactose-fermenting organisms of Escherichia coli.*

Fig. 2.19 *Cytopathic effect of respiratory syncytial virus (RSV) in tissue culture.*

TISSUE CULTURE

Viruses are pathogens that are obligate intracellular parasites requiring living cells or tissues in order to be propagated. Monolayers of cells are inoculated, maintained and examined for evidence of a cytopathic effect. The specific cell line and cytopathic effect help to differentiate classes of viruses. The ability to detect viruses by antigen staining, the cytopathic effect they produce, and direct or indirect immunofluorescence using immunological methods are commonly used laboratory methods for detecting viruses. An example of the cytopathic effect of respiratory syncytial virus (RSV) is shown in **Figure 2.19**. An example of immunofluorescence for RSV is shown in **Figure 2.20**.

MOLECULAR TECHNIQUES

There are a number of techniques that employ molecular methods to detect pathogens directly or to quantify the number of organisms present. The most common techniques include:
- the polymerase chain reaction;
- the ligase chain reaction; and
- the use of branched-chain detection of deoxyribonucleic acid (DNA) or ribose nucleic acid (RNA).

The basis of these methods is the use of DNA or RNA extracted from patients' specimens, which is then mixed with primers which can replicate the nucleic acid of the organism of interest. Using very high temperatures to melt the nucleic acids, heat-stable polymerases allow the primers to synthesise complementary copies of the DNA or RNA of interest.

There are a number of variations on this theme that allow very high copy numbers of small quantities of pathogens to be detected. Even pathogens that are very difficult to cultivate, such as the organism that causes Whipple's disease, have been able to be characterized by the use of the polymerase chain reaction. The ligase chain reaction is used to detect *Chlamydia trachomatis* and *N. gonorrhoeae* in cervical specimens or urine specimens. It has been shown to be more sensitive and specific than culture methods or enzyme detection methods. The branched chain DNA replication methods are used to test blood samples for pathogens such as the human immunodeficiency virus (HIV) and hepatitis C virus in order to quantify the amount of pathogen present. These tests are

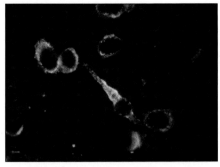

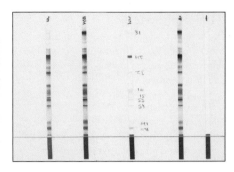

Fig. 2.20 *Direct immunofluorescence of nasal secretions from an infant with RSV bronchiolitis.*

Fig. 2.21 *Western blot from patient with HIV infection.*

referred to as measurements of 'viral load'. Other methods, such as the use of immunoblots, can detect various proteins made by the organisms. An example is the use of a 'Western blot' to detect HIV proteins (**Fig. 2.21**). Such blots are employed routinely to confirm infection with HIV.

SEROLOGICAL METHODS

An organism may elaborate a specific antigen or series of antigenic components that are able to be detected in serum, plasma or other body fluids or secretions. These antigen detection methods using enzyme immunoassays have formed the basis for detection of *C. trachomatis* in cervical secretions, *Legionella pneumophila* in the urine, or cryptococcal or histoplasmal antigen in cerebrospinal fluid.

Indirect detection looking for evidence of antibody development can also be employed. For example, antibody to Epstein–Barr virus may demonstrate a past infection. By using methods to separate immunoglobulin M from immunoglobulin G, it may be possible to differentiate recent infection from past infection. Many antibody detection methods are available for the detection of infection with viruses, including HIV, measles virus, rubella virus and cytomegalovirus.

Organisms may be distinguished by serological typing of strains. For example, *E. coli* 0157/H7 has particular pathogenic potential owing to toxins that it produces. Infection with this strain causes bloody diarrhoea, which may progress to the haemolytic–uremic syndrome. Taking an emulsion of colonies from the agar, and typing with specific antiserum will enable the laboratory to document infection with this specific serotype. Another example of typing is a specific agglutination reaction with typing serum to differentiate group A β-haemolytic streptococci from other streptococci.

BIOCHEMICAL TESTING

There are a number of biochemical schemes that can help differentiate organisms from one another. There are some simple methods that differentiate some organisms easily and that are useful to know.

The catalase test

For example, the ability of an emulsion of organisms to produce gas when exposed to hydrogen peroxide by bubbling to produce water and oxygen (the catalase test) differentiates staphylococci (which are catalase-positive) from streptococci (which are catalase-negative).

The coagulase test

S. aureus, a significant pathogen, can be differentiated from nonpathogenic staphylococci by the ability to coagulate fibrinogen. The so-called coagulase test takes an emulsified organism and adds plasma (coagulase) to it on a slide or inoculated in a tube (**Fig. 2.22**). The ability to coagulate the plasma defines virtually all strains of *S. aureus*.

Other biochemical tests

The differentiation of streptococci can be accomplished by a few biochemical tests *S. pneumoniae* can be easily differentiated from other streptococci by its sensitivity to chemicals like optochin (ethyl hydrocupreine) (**Fig. 2.23**) or by the dissolution of colonies that occurs when bile salts are added to a plate where colonies are growing (the so-called bile solubility test) (**Fig. 2.24**).

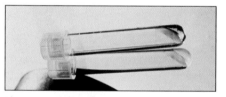

Fig. 2.22 *Tube coagulase test showing presence of* Staphylococcus aureus.

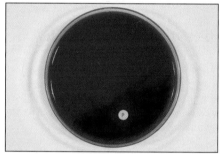

Fig. 2.23 Streptococcus pneumoniae *on an agar plate showing sensitivity to ethyl hydrocupreine (optochin).*

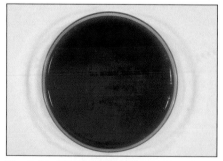

Fig. 2.24 *Bile solubility of colonies of* Streptococcus pneumoniae.

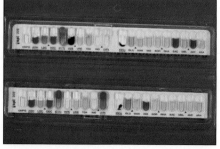

Fig. 2.25 *Biochemical reactions of the API test kit.*

There are a number of tests that can differentiate other species of organisms, and many of these biochemical tests are incorporated into commercial test kits that use 15–30 different biochemicals. Examples include kits such as the API test kit (manufactured by Bio-Merieux) (**Fig. 2.25**) and the Antimicrobic Test System (manufactured by Vitek). Discussion of all of the biochemical test methods available is beyond the scope of this text.

ANTIMICROBIAL SENSITIVITY TESTING

The laboratory plays an important role in the management of infections by providing information about the susceptibility of microbes to antimicrobial agents, through the use of antimicrobial sensitivity testing. Organisms may be sensitive or resistant to the antimicrobial agent. Organisms are considered susceptible if the level of sensitivity is such that therapy with a given agent is likely to be successful.

There are a number of methods that can detect the level of sensitivity of a given organism to an antimicrobial agent. Some methods employ broth dilution techniques, in which the organism is grown in broth and tested against varying concentrations of an antimicrobial agent. These methods can document the minimal concentration of the drug necessary to inhibit growth, the minimal inhibitory concentration (MIC). Both broth dilution and microbroth dilution techniques are available to test organisms to a panel of drugs that are likely to have activity (**Fig. 2.26**).

The lowest quantity of drug necessary to kill (as opposed to inhibit) the organism is defined as that concentration necessary to reduce growth by 99.9% (i.e. 3 logs of growth); this is the minimum bactericidal concentration (MBC). Typically this is determined by

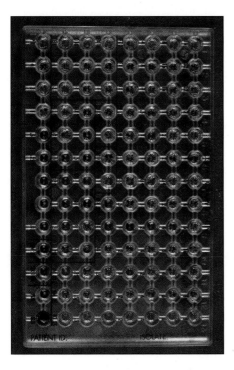

Fig. 2.26 *Microbroth dilution sensitivity test panel.*

subculturing the organism from the broth cultures with different concentrations of the antimicrobial agent and then examining the overnight cultures for growth. A drug that is capable of 99.9% reduction in growth is called bactericidal. Antimicrobials with bactericidal capability are necessary to treat certain infections, such as bacterial endocarditis or bacterial meningitis. All such testing is based on a standardized inoculum of the organism and the use of achievable and nontoxic concentrations of the antimicrobial agent in humans.

There are available a number of automated or semiautomated methods of antimicrobial sensitivity testing, which employ panels of drugs to be tested. Most use microbroth dilution techniques, in which wells with predetermined quantities of drug are inoculated with standard quantities of the organism. Such methods typically provide only MIC data. Another method commonly used in the USA is the Kirby–Bauer method. Discs with standard concentrations of an antimicrobial agent are layered onto an agar plate that has been inoculated with micro-organisms. The size of the zone of inhibition around the disc is defined as indicating susceptibility or resistance for each drug (**Fig. 2.27**). The actual MIC cannot be determined with this method but drug susceptibility can be.

For fastidious organisms, agar with antibiotics incorporated into it can be used. Organisms can be inoculated onto the agar and observed for growth after overnight incubation. Agar dilution techniques can be used to screen for susceptibility for large numbers of micro-organisms. Another method, which has become very popular, is the epsillometer test (E test). An inoculum of organisms is placed on an agar plate. The 'E strip', which contains a concentration dependent gradient of antibiotic, is placed on the inoculum. After an incubation of 18–24 hours, the intersection of growth with the concentration can be read as the MIC (**Fig. 2.28**). This test method is particularly useful for testing more fastidious organisms, such as *S. pneumoniae*.

The methods for detecting the sensitivity of viruses, fungi and parasites to chemotherapeutic agents are much less standardized than the methods used for bacteria. This is largely due to the complexity of their life cycles, different growth characteristics and problems with testing in varying media. Techniques that use genetically engineered probes to look for resistance elements in bacteria, viruses and parasites are under development.

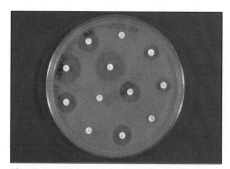

Fig. 2.27 *Kirby–Bauer sensitivity test plate.*

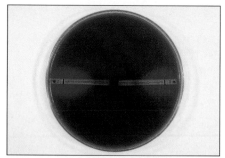

Fig. 2.28 *E test plate showing minimum inhibitory concentration for* Streptococcus pneumoniae.

chapter 3

Hospital-Acquired Infections

Approximately 5% of all patients develop an infection during their stay in the hospital. These hospital-acquired infections are known as nosocomial infections. An infection that is the result of intervention by a physician, in or out of a hospital, is known as an iatrogenic infection. Nosocomial infections often result in prolongation of hospital stay and are extraordinarily costly in terms of morbidity and even mortality. It is estimated that about $US 5 billion is spent each year in the USA for the management of hospital-acquired infections.

A number of factors related to hospitalization predispose patients to the risk of a hospital-acquired infection. The most important ones are those that violate the host's own defenses. Invasive procedures produce new portals of entry for micro-organisms from the patient's own flora or from the environment. Examples of this are the use of devices such as endotracheal tubes, mechanical ventilators, intravenous or intra-arterial catheters, and any surgical procedures.

Broadly speaking, the frequency of development of nosocomial infections is directly related to the severity of the underlying disease (i.e. patients who have a high likelihood of dying during their hospitalization also run a higher risk of developing a nosocomial infection; in contrast, patients who are admitted with less severe disease have a lesser chance of acquiring infections in the hospital). This underscores the need for improved management of the severely compromised patient. Unfortunately, it is estimated that only about one-third to one-half of all nosocomial infections are preventable under the most favourable conditions.

AGENTS OF NOSOCOMIAL AND IATROGENIC INFECTIONS

Virtually any micro-organism can cause a nosocomial infection. Often the most common causative agents may not be especially pathogenic; in fact, sometimes they may be even less pathogenic than those that cause disease outside hospital. However, given an immunocompromised patient, these organisms become important pathogens.

BACTERIA

Many of the important nosocomial pathogens have evolved as a result of antibiotic exposure. One example is *Enterobacter* spp. These organisms are among the leaders as a cause of nosocomial infection. Yet 25 years ago they were considered to be plant pathogens and only very rarely pathogenic in humans. The inherent resistance of *Enterobacter* spp. to first generation cephalosporin antibiotics as well as their presence in normal flora has enabled these organisms to develop an ecological niche within the hospital.

Gram-negative bacterial strains that possess plasmid-mediated, multiple antibiotic resistance are also commonly encountered in nosocomial infections. Plasmid transfer occurs among different strains of the same species and even among different genera. Transfer of antibiotic resistance between organisms has been demonstrated in catheterized patients (Foley catheters) between bacteria in the urine. Transfer has been demonstrated to occur between organisms on the skin of the same patient. Presumably, transfer of antibiotic resistance takes place in the gastrointestinal tract as well. Antibiotic-resistant pathogens have become so common that methicillin-resistant *Staphylococcus aureus*, aminoglycoside-resistant and cephalosporin-resistant Gram-negative bacteria are regularly encountered in nosocomial infections, and now vancomycin-resistant and ampicillin-resistant enterococci are being encountered as well. A list of common nosocomial pathogens is detailed in **Figure 3.1**.

VIRUSES

There are also a number of viruses that are important as causes of nosocomial infection (**Fig. 3.2**). Respiratory syncytial virus (RSV) is an important cause of nosocomial infection among neonates with congenital heart disease and bronchopulmonary dysplasia (**Fig. 3.3**). It has become a recognized and serious cause of pneumonia in both paediatric and adult bone marrow transplant recipients. Diagnosis can be made by direct or indirect immunofluorescence of nasal washings (**see Fig 2.21**) or bronchoalveolar lavage. Another common viral pathogen is rotavirus, which causes epidemic diarrhoeal illness in nurseries. Rotavirus can be diagnosed by an enzyme immunoassay test of stool.

Common pathogens in nosocomial infections	Viruses of importance in nosocomial infection
Staphylococcus aureus	Respiratory syncytial virus (RSV)
Pseudomonas aeruginosa	Varicella-zoster virus
Staphylococcus epidermidis	Cytomegalovirus
Enterococcus spp.	Influenza virus
Escherichia coli	Measles virus
Klebsiella pneumoniae	Rubella virus
Enterobacter spp.	Rotavirus
Candida spp.	Hepatitis A virus, hepatitis B virus, hepatitis C virus
	Adenovirus
	Parainfluenza virus

Fig. 3.1 *Common pathogens in nosocomial infections.*

Fig. 3.2 *Viruses of importance in nosocomial infection.*

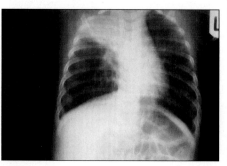

Fig. 3.3 *Chest X-ray of child with respiratory syncytial virus infection.*

Cytomegalovirus is an important nosocomial pathogen complicating organ transplantation. This organism is discussed in greater detail in Chapter 13.

A number of other viral pathogens may cause hospital-acquired infection, including influenza virus, measles virus, rubella, and varicella-zoster virus. These viruses have the potential to spread readily because one means of transmission for each is by the respiratory route.

TRANSMISSION IN HOSPITAL

A hospital is a microenvironment in which organisms can be transferred in a variety of ways from one person to another, including from hospital staff to patients (**Fig. 3.4**).

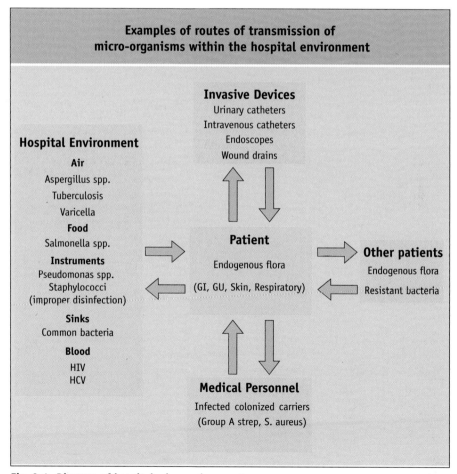

Fig. 3.4 *Diagram of hospital microenvironment.*

Transmission between persons may be direct, by hand contact, or indirect, by inhalation, ingestion or puncture through the integument (**Fig. 3.5**). Examples include infections due to methicillin-resistant staphylococci, which spread directly between patients or via hospital personnel. Tubercle bacilli are transmitted through aerosolization and inhalation. Viral agents, such as those of varicella or influenza, may be spread through the air to susceptible immunocompromised patients. Blood used for transfusions may be contaminated with hepatitis viruses A, B and C, or the human immunodeficiency virus. Food handlers may contaminate food eaten by patients. Physicians and nurses may introduce micro-organisms into deeper tissues during operations or while dressing surgical or other wounds.

Unusual epidemics can sometimes be traced to specific carriers among members of the hospital staff. For example, well-documented epidemics caused by group A β-hemolytic streptococci have been attributed to carriers who had contact with patients in the operating room. In one epidemic, the organisms were located in the carrier's vagina, from where they were presumably aerosolized through normal body movements.

Micro-organisms that spread to patients may be endemic to the hospital environment. Notable examples include the fungi that cause aspergillosis, which may be present as more or less visible mildew on the walls of moist rooms or construction panels. Infections by exogenous organisms may also be acquired from improperly sterilized surgical instruments and even contaminated disinfectant solutions. Fortunately, these are rare events in a proper hospital setting.

Examples of routes of transmission of hospital infection

Route	Organism	Site or type of infection
Airborne	Mycobacterium tuberculosis	Pneumonia
	Legionella spp.	Pneumonia
	Aspergillus spp.	Pneumonia
	Varicella-zoster virus	Pneumonia
Droplet spread	Influenza virus	Pneumonia
	Respiratory Syncytial virus	Bronchiolitis
	Group A, β-hemolytic streptococci	Wound, skin
Direct contact	Staphyloccus aureus	Surgical wound, cutaneous
	Group A, β-hemolytic Streptococci	Surgical wound
Indirect contact (via object)	Pseudomonas spp.	Urinary tract, ventilator
Common vehicle	Salmonella spp.	Gastrointestinal tract (via food or carrier)
	Campylobacter spp.	Gastrointestinal tract (via food or carrier)
	Hepatitis A	Gastrointestinal tract (via food or carrier), blood (transmission)
	Hepatitis B	Blood, contaminated instruments

Fig. 3.5 *Examples of routes of transmission of hospital infection.*

Patients acquire nosocomial infections as the result of breaks in their own defences and from their inability to combat infection (**Fig. 3.6**). These breaks usually occur as the result of invasive diagnostic or therapeutic interventions that physicians perform on their patients. For these reasons, the most common nosocomial infections affect the urinary tract, because catheterization of the bladder is frequently used with bedridden patients. The commonly used Foley catheter bypasses the normal mucosal barriers and facilitates the entry of organisms that colonize the skin or the urinary introitus. The next most frequent type of infection is that of surgical wounds, followed by respiratory tract infections. A diagram of the relative proportion of major hospital infections by site is shown in **Figure 3.7**.

Common hospital acquired infections and frequently associated organisms

Type of infection	Most common organism
Surgical wound infection	*Staphylococcus aureus*
	Escherichia coli
	Enterococcus faecalis
Pneumonia	*Klebsiella pneumoniae*
	Pseudomonas aeruginosa
	Staphylococcus aureus
	Enterobacter spp.
	Escherichia coli
Intravenous catheter infection	*Staphylococcus epidermidis*
	Staphylococcus aureus
	Enterococcus faecalis
	Candida spp.
Urinary catheter infection	*Escherichia coli*
	Enterococcus faecalis
	Pseudomonas aeruginosa
	Klebsiella spp.

Fig. 3.6 *Common hospital acquired infections and frequently associated organisms.*

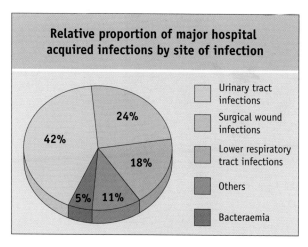

Relative proportion of major hospital acquired infections by site of infection

42%
24%
18%
5%
11%

Urinary tract infections

Surgical wound infections

Lower respiratory tract infections

Others

Bacteraemia

Fig. 3.7 *Relative proportion of major hospital acquired infections by site of infection.*

The skin barrier is breached by the use of intravenous catheters or devices used to measure intravascular pressure. The longer intravenous catheters remain in place, the higher the risk for both local infection and bacteraemia. This underscores the need for vigilance in the care of patients with indwelling devices. According to national surveys in the USA, the rate of nosocomial bacteremia almost doubled in the 1980s, and that due to this *Staphylococcus epidermidis* tripled. In intravenous therapy, there are many different areas, from the bottle to the intravenous catheter, where contamination may occur. The risk of intravenous catheter-related infection is generally influenced by the type of catheter and the duration of catheterization. Patients who have large-bore catheters that require surgical insertion have the highest risk. The diagnosis of intravascular catheter infection can be made by removal of the device with culture by semiquantitative methodology, using a 'roll-plate' technique (**Fig. 3.8**). This method distinguishes significant versus insignificant colonization. The usual pathogens tend to be *S. aureus*, *S. epidermidis*, a variety of Gram-negative rods or *Candida* spp. Patients with a chronic need for intravenous access (e.g. a hemodialysis, fistula or catheter) are particularly susceptible (**Fig. 3.9**).

Another example of the role of the normal skin in protecting the host from microbial invasion is seen in burn victims. Frequently, patients who have extensive second- or third-degree burns become colonized with bacteria, especially *Pseudomonas aeruginosa*. Necrotizing lesions at the site of skin damage are accompanied by sepsis, the major cause of death in burn victims.

The most common risk factor for the development of nosocomial pneumonia is the use of an endotracheal tube. This bypasses the normal airway defenses and allows the entry of organisms into the airway. In the early 1960s, when mechanical ventilation of the lungs was being developed, it was recognized that epidemics of Gram-negative pneumonia occurred because nebulized mists contained bacteria-laden aerosols. An understanding of the problem brought about changes in design, which have virtually eliminated the ventilator as a source of hospital-acquired pneumonia (**Fig. 3.10**). Nosocomial pneumonia may be difficult to detect because patients in the intensive care unit are frequently colonized with Gram-negative rods (**Fig. 3.11**), yet pulmonary infiltrates due to acute respiratory distress syndrome may be caused by a noninfectious etiology. Patients with endotracheal tubes still develop pneumonia, but now the offending organisms tend to come from the patient's stomach or intestine and colonize the nasopharynx. From here, they may become aspirated

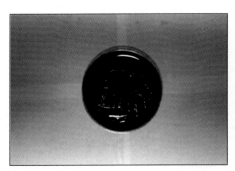

Fig. 3.8 *An example of roll-plate technique showing* Pseudomonas aeruginosa *from a TPN catheter.*

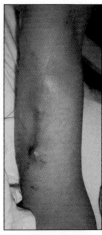

Fig. 3.9 *Patient with haemodialysis fistula infected with* Pseudomonas aeruginosa.

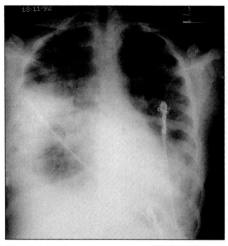

Fig. 3.11 *Sputum Gram stain of Gram-negative organisms in a patient only colonized with organisms. Note the absence of polymorphonuclear leucocytes.*

Fig. 3.10 *Chest X-ray of a patient with nosocomial pneumonia.*

into the lungs. Other examples of nosocomial infections acquired by inhalation can be seen in hospital epidemics of influenza and varicella, which are particularly troublesome for immunocompromised patients.

Epidemics of nosocomial infection sometimes result from the ingestion of pathogenic bacteria. The organisms are often those associated with community-acquired infections, such as *Salmonella* spp., hepatitis A virus and rotavirus; rotavirus is most commonly seen among neonates or infants. Epidemics of salmonellosis in hospitals usually result from eating foods contaminated during preparation. They have also resulted from the use of contaminated animal products used for diagnostic purposes, such as carmine dye.

The complexity of a hospital environment provides innumerable opportunities for the encounter of patients with micro-organisms. Some of these are specific for the hospital environment and are not usually found elsewhere. An example is the use of contaminated intravenous solutions, which have caused many epidemics. Contamination rarely takes place at the point of manufacture; more commonly, it occurs during the handling of bottles and infusion lines.

Instruments and dressings that have been improperly sterilized before surgery also provide a possible source of infection. A whole technology has developed around the problems of determining if autoclaves and sterilizing ovens perform their expected task. Thus, it is customary to insert a vial containing bacterial spores with the material to be autoclaved, and to determine spore viability afterward. Deviation from established procedures may well result in improper sterilization and in contamination of surgical or other wounds.

Surgical wound infections are the most costly of all nosocomial infections. Some are clearly preventable. They are frequently due to *S. aureus*, but may be mixed aerobic and anaerobic flora as well (**Fig. 3.12**).

Primary bacteraemia is defined as bacteraemia that cannot be ascribed to another focus of infection. Often, primary bacteraemia is either the result of a contaminated intravenous line or associated with granulocytopenia in the immunosuppressed leukaemic patient.

25

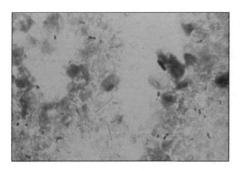

Fig. 3.12 *Gram stain from surgical wound infection due to mixed aerobic–anaerobic flora.*

Another example of primary bacteraemia is generally seen in leukaemia or lymphoma patients who are granulocytopenic as a result of cancer chemotherapy. Patients will frequently become bacteraemic, primarily from an intestinal focus. The usual pathogens in this setting are Gram-negative rods, which may originate from the patient's endogenous flora or may be exogenously acquired in the hospital.

Nosocomial aspergillosis, although not common, has recently been seen more often among immunosuppressed patients. A number of reported epidemics have been linked to hospital construction and contamination of air conditioning systems. Large numbers of fungal spores in the air lead to nasal or bronchial colonization. Immunosuppression and the resultant granulocytopenia, along with broad-spectrum antibacterial antibiotics, help the organism become established in the airways.

Another aspect of hospital infection that has received prominence recently has been the risk of transmission by needle-stick injury of hepatitis B and C viruses and the human immunodeficiency virus (HIV) to health-care workers. Foremost among the ways of preventing needle-stick injuries is the common-sense avoidance of recapping needles, which accounts for 30% of these injuries. Hepatitis B can be prevented by vaccination, which should be given to all health workers. However, needle-stick transmission of hepatitis C virus and HIV can still occur, and, for the unaware, hepatitis B still poses a problem. Fortunately there is evidence that use of prompt antiretroviral therapy can prevent needle-stick transmission of HIV and early intervention is important to prevent the spread of this virus.

CONTROL

There are a number of approaches to the control and prevention of hospital-acquired infection. The major preventive strategy is the interruption of transmission from patient to patient. Included in this strategy is surveillance for infected patients and isolation of infected patients. Additional strategies are boosting the host's immunity to infection, the use of appropriate antibiotics for prophylaxis in high-risk situations such as surgery, prompt recognition and treatment of infection and removal of invasive devices as early as possible.

STERILIZATION AND DISINFECTION
Another facet to the prevention of hospital acquired infection is effective disinfection and sterilization. Sterile items are free from all viable organisms; disinfection refers to the removal of most but not all viable organisms. Sterilization can be achieved through heat, irradiation or chemicals. Moist heat in the form of steam under pressure forms the basis for autoclaving materials.

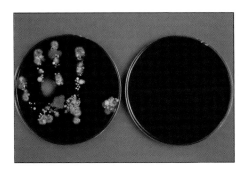

Fig. 3.13 *The effect of hand washing on removal of organisms from hands.*

Control of nosocomial infections requires awareness by all health-care professionals. Hand washing between patient contacts is a simple but much-neglected procedure. It can decrease transmission of micro-organisms between hospital staff and patients. **Figure 3.13** shows the effect of hand washing on the carriage of microbial flora. The use of aseptic techniques during surgical and other invasive procedures, as stressed in surgical training, significantly prevents these infections.

Hospitals have instituted infection control committees, whose responsibility it is to oversee all aspects of infection control within the institution. They supervise surveillance of hospital-acquired infections, establish policies and procedures to prevent such infections, and have the power to intervene when necessary in investigations of epidemics or other problems. Most hospitals have specific personnel (infection control practitioners or infection control 'sisters'), who are assigned these tasks and function as the 'eyes and ears' of the committee. These infection control practitioners are responsible for tracing epidemics, monitoring the infection rate and determining the level of isolation of patients. Of course, intense efforts are invested in trying to prevent infections in the increasing number of immunocompromised hosts and in working out effective means to prevent nosocomial infections.

chapter 4

Principles of Epidemiology

INTRODUCTION

Epidemiology is the study of the determinants of disease in a population. It deals with both infectious and noninfectious aetiologies. When infectious agents are involved, the aim is to understand their mode of transmission and the predisposition of a population to a particular agent.

The practical purpose of epidemiology is to control the spread of disease in a population, either by limiting microbial transmission or by altering the susceptibility of a population. Commonly used measures include:
- removing the source of the agent;
- controlling its transmission; and
- immunizing the population.

'Infection' is the term that indicates the presence of an infectious agent in a population whereas 'disease' is the term used when there are clinical symptoms and signs. Many infectious diseases are communicable (e.g. measles, polio, tuberculosis). Others, such as a ruptured appendix, urinary tract infections and osteomyelitis, are not.

INCUBATION PERIOD

From an epidemiological perspective an important determinant for an agent is the incubation period of a disease (i.e. the time interval from exposure to the agent to the development of disease). The length of the incubation period differs considerably among infectious diseases, from a few hours to months or years. It is influenced by many factors. For example, a large infective dose may shorten it and a small infective dose may lengthen it.

To the epidemiologist, the incubation period is particularly important because, during this time, some diseases may be transmitted from asymptomatic patients. Control of transmission may, therefore, have to rely on special surveillance methods that are able to locate infected but asymptomatic persons.

The periods of incubation and of communicability are not always the same. For example, the incubation period in hepatitis A most commonly lasts for 2–4 weeks; however, infected people can transmit the virus for only 1 week before the onset of the disease and for a very brief period (usually less than 1 week) after the onset of disease.

The period of communicability in some infectious diseases may extend itself long after the symptoms of the disease abate, as in the case of a chronic asymptomatic carrier. For example, a carrier of hepatitis B virus can usually transmit the virus for the whole period of carriage. Carriers of *Salmonella typhi* may carry organisms for months or years in the stool. Examples of incubation periods for a number of agents are listed in **Figure 4.1**.

29

Incubation periods for several infectious agents		
Agent	Median incubation period (days)	Range (days)
Hepatitis A virus	28	14–42
Hepatitis B virus	60	30–180
Epstein-Barr virus	21	28–42
Mycoplasma pneumoniae	14	7–21
Measles virus	10	8–13
Rubella virus	18	12–23
Varicella-zoster virus	14	9–21
Human immunodeficiency virus	60	30–180
Bordetella pertussis	7	5–21
Respiratory syncytial virus	5	2–8

Fig. 4.1 *Incubation periods for several infectious agents.*

MODE OF SPREAD

Another characteristic of an agent is the mode by which it is spread. The mode of transmission (Fig. 4.2) may be:
* vertical (i.e. the passage of an agent from an infected mother to her fetus or infant); or
* horizontal (i.e. from person to person, as among individuals in a household).

Organisms associated with various modes of transmission	
Mode of transmission	Examples of organism
Respiratory	Influenza virus *Mycoplasma* spp. Varicella-zoster virus
Sexual	*Neisseria gonorrhoeae* Human immunodeficiency virus (HIV) *Treponema pallidum* (syphilis)
Faecal-oral	Hepatitis A virus *Salmonella* spp.
Blood-borne	Hepatitis B virus Hepatitis C virus HIV
Vector-borne	*Borellia burgdorferi* (Lyme disease) *Rickettsia rickettsii* (Rocky Mountain spotted fever) *Plasmodium* spp. (malaria)
Vertical (materno-fetal)	*Toxoplasma gondii* Cytomegalovirus Hepatitis B virus HIV

Fig. 4.2 *Organisms associated with various modes of transmission.*

VERTICAL TRANSMISSION

The most intimate mode is via the transplacental route. Examples of such congenitally acquired diseases are syphilis, rubella (**Fig. 4.3**) and toxoplasmosis (**Fig. 4.4**). Newborn babies may also pick up chlamydiae, gonococci, cytomegalovirus, hepatitis B virus or the human immunodeficiency virus (HIV) during passage through the birth canal. Some of these organisms may be transmitted via mother's milk.

HORIZONTAL TRANSMISSION

Horizontal transmission generally occurs between people in close proximity, and includes intimate modes, such as sexual intercourse, or more casual ones, such as touching another person or breathing of aerosols. The actual path of an organism from one person to another depends on the way the agent exits the body of the donor. Thus, bacteria or viruses that infect the respiratory tract are often expelled as aerosols during coughing and even talking, and may be inhaled by bystanders. If the organism is resistant to drying, as is the case with the tubercle bacillus, the danger of inhalation may persist for a long time. Some diseases are acquired through traumatic breaches of the skin or mucous membranes, such as from an insect bite (e.g. Lyme disease). Many of the agents that are transmitted by insect vectors have different life cycles in the vector and in the host. Blood-borne pathogens, such as hepatitis B virus, hepatitis C virus and HIV, can be transmitted through the transfused blood itself or by needle stick. Note that some of these organisms may be transmitted by more than one of these routes. Thus, HIV infection may be passed transplacentally, by sexual intercourse, by the use of needles or by blood transfusion.

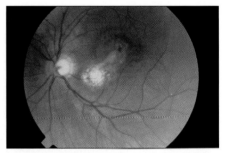

Fig. 4.4 *Retinal changes caused by congenital toxoplasmosis.*

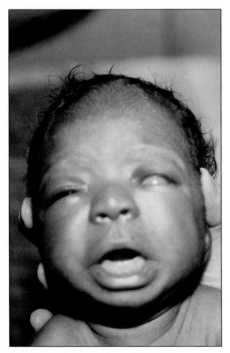

Fig. 4.3 *Glaucoma in a child with congenital rubella.*

OTHER MODES OF TRANSMISSION

A number of infectious agents are acquired from nonhuman reservoirs. These include the zoonoses, in which the reservoir is an animal. Transmission from the animal may be direct, as in the bite from a rabid dog (**Fig. 4.5**), or via insect vectors, such as transmission of *Yersinia pestis* (the organism that causes plague), viral encephalitides or the newly described Hantavirus. Lyme disease is also a zoonosis in which the natural reservoir is mammals such as deer who share ticks (*Ixodes dammini*) (**Fig. 4.6**) with humans.

Another means of transmission is contact with a contaminated environment, such as with rodent excreta infected with Hantavirus. The nature of the vector and the organism may vary throughout the world. For example, the presence of malaria is due to the mosquito species capable of supporting transmission (**Fig. 4.7**). Furthermore, the presence of drug resistance to *Plasmodium falciparum* is limited to certain parts of the world (**Fig. 4.8**). It is incumbent upon physicians who prescribe prophylaxis to know the distribution of these infections. Examples of geographically restricted diseases are the presence of *Histoplasma capsulatum* in the Mississippi River valley of the USA (**Fig. 4.9**), the distribution of *Schistosoma japonicum* in South East Asia, the presence of *Clonorchis sinensis* in China.

For other diseases, the reservoir is the inanimate environment, and the organisms live freely in nature. For example, the clostridia of gas gangrene are commonly found in soil. However, even in such cases, humans or animals may contribute to the frequency with which the agents are found in nature. For instance, cholera bacilli grow naturally in warm estuaries, probably on the surface of shellfish. However, contamination from human faeces may help the organisms become established in a previously uninfected area.

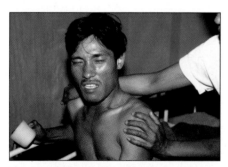

Fig. 4.5 *Hydrophobic rabies in a patient from Thailand.*

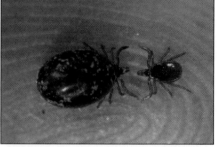

Fig. 4.6 **Ixodes dammini** *(deer ticks): Examples of a non-fed nymph and a replete nymph are shown on a fingertip. Courtesy of Richard J. Pollack, PhD.*

Fig. 4.7 **Anophyles mosquito** *(Anophyles gambiae s.1.) feeding on a hand. Courtesy of Richard J. Pollack, PhD.*

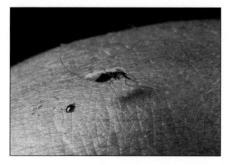

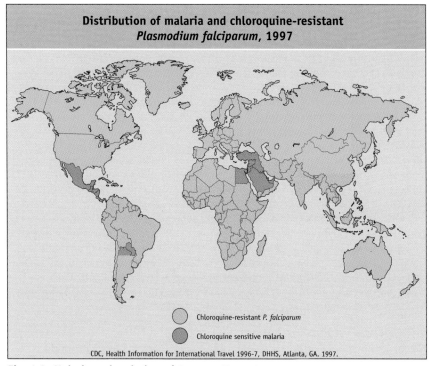

Fig. 4.8 *Malaria and malaria-resistance patterns.*

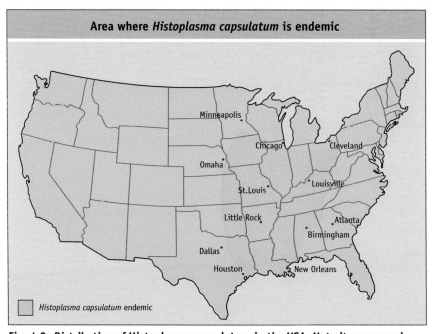

Fig. 4.9 *Distribution of* Histoplasma capsulatum *in the USA. Note its presence in the Mississippi River Valley delta.*

HOST SUSCEPTIBILITY

Human beings differ in their predisposition to infectious diseases. We have all encountered individuals who seem more prone to respiratory or intestinal infections than the majority. For many of these persons, we do not know the reason for this susceptibility. They may have subtle deficiencies in certain of their defense mechanisms. When these deficiencies become severe and the risks are more evident, the cause is often easier to ascertain.

The epidemiologist must be aware of the different susceptibility of members of the population. Age, sex, nutritional status, previous exposure and immune competence all contribute to a greater or lesser susceptibility to a particular infectious disease. Thus, children and older persons are frequently more susceptible to bacterial pneumonia or intestinal infections. The incidence of the carrier state of hepatitis B virus is greater in males than in females. It is also more frequent among people with Down's syndrome or those receiving haemodialysis.

Genetic factors are also known to play a role, although for the most part, the data are inconclusive. The importance of these factors is often difficult to unravel from a myriad of socioeconomic factors, such as those that contribute to the state of health and nutrition. Nonetheless, the role of genetic factors has been well established in certain diseases. One of the most intensively studied genetic effects is the decreased susceptibility to malaria of persons with the sickle cell trait. It is also well established that non-Caucasians are more prone to the disseminated form of coccidioidomycosis than Caucasians.

IMMUNIZATION

Epidemiologists and public health officials can reduce the host susceptibility of the population through the use of active immunization.

Active immunization

Active immunization boosts the host's own immune response to make antibodies. Live, attenuated and killed vaccines are used for this purpose. A compendium of available vaccines is listed in **Figure 4.10**. Examples of diseases that have been virtually eliminated through the use of vaccination include polio, congenital rubella, small pox and infection with *Haemophilus influenzae* type B. Improved immunogenicity of vaccines should increase host immunity to a number of additional agents.

When immunization is successful it may last a lifetime and confer 'herd immunity' or protection to the unimmunized cohort by preventing the entry of the agent into the susceptible population.

Passive immunization

Another form of immunization is passive immunization. This form of prophylaxis utilizes the administration of antibodies to previously unimmunized people. The antibodies will not persist but will provide short-term protection. Use of gammaglobulin for household contacts of patients infected with hepatitis A virus is one example of passive immunization.

Agents and diseases for which active immunization is available	
Diphtheria	Haemophilus influenzae
Pertussis	Streptococcus pneumoniae
Tetanus	Influenza
Polio	Varicella
Measles	Hepatitis B
Mumps	Neisseria meningitidis
Rubella	Smallpox

Fig. 4.10 *Agents and diseases for which active immunization is available.*

EPIDEMICS

An epidemic investigation is undertaken when there is an increase in the number of cases of a disease over what is considered to be the norm or standard. The determination of an epidemic depends solely on the background incidence of the disease in the population and not on an absolute cut-off point. For example, before the advent of the polio vaccine in the 1950s, there were about 50,000 cases of the disease in the USA annually. After the vaccine came into widespread use, the number of cases dropped dramatically to about 10 per year. Therefore, two cases of polio might be considered to be an epidemic!

In addition to epidemics, there are endemic and pandemic diseases. An endemic infectious disease is one that is consistently found in the population, such as dental caries, gonorrhoea or athlete's foot. A pandemic is a worldwide epidemic; examples are the current AIDS pandemic and the Spanish flu pandemic of 1918–1919.

CONCLUSIONS

In a civilized society, epidemiology is everyone's business because of the impact of diseases on public health. The practising physician and all the members of the health-care team must be aware of the public health implications of a given patient's infectious disease. To safeguard both the public interest and the rights of privacy of patients, a considerable body of local and national laws has been developed in most countries of the world. For instance, in the USA and the UK, a number of communicable diseases are classed as 'notifiable' – that is, physicians are obliged to report them to the relevant public health authority. The information collected is published in a readily available pamphlet: in the USA, in the *Morbidity and Mortality Weekly Reports* (MMWR); in the UK, in the *Communicable Disease Report* (CDR). These reports list all routine information and call attention to unusual occurrences. In addition, each local city and town has its own surveillance mechanism and reporting requirements for the study of communicable diseases within its borders. Reference laboratories are equipped to carry out special diagnostic tests that are often outside the scope of hospital laboratories.

Epidemiology may appear to be a remote discipline practised mainly by public health officials. In fact, it pervades all forms of medical practice and furnishes important clues for the diagnosis of infectious diseases. Thus, inquiry into time and place characteristics should be part of the usual process of taking a clinical history. Epidemiological information can reveal how people encounter disease agents and can help reduce exposure to and spread of infectious diseases.

chapter 5

Cardiovascular Infection

ENDOCARDITIS

Infectious endocarditis usually refers to infection of the heart valves caused by bacteria and fungi. Vascular endothelium elsewhere in the body may also become infected and produce a similar clinical picture, known as endovascular infection. Endocarditis is usually classified as infection occurring either on native valves or on prosthetic heart valves.

NATIVE-VALVE ENDOCARDITIS

About 80% of patients who develop native-valve endocarditis have some pre-existing valvular lesion. In the past, this was usually caused by rheumatic heart disease. Now, more common abnormalities include congenitally bicuspid aortic valves, mitral valve prolapse and degenerative, calcified, sclerotic aortic valves. The mitral valve is the most commonly affected, followed by the aortic and then tricuspid valves. Infection of the pulmonary valve is exceedingly rare. Congenital heart defects, except atrial septal defects, predispose the patient to endocarditis.

The causes of native valve endocarditis are listed in **Figure 5.1**. Viridans streptococci continue to be the main pathogens but their relative importance may be declining. These organisms are part of the normal oral flora; hence the association of endocarditis with poor dentition. Endocarditis caused by *Streptococcus bovis* is highly associated with colonic neoplasia, so the finding of this organism in the blood should prompt a search for a colonic polyp or carcinoma. Enterococcal infections (*Enterococcus faecalis* and *Enterococcus*

Fig. 5.1 *Causes of native-valve endocarditis.*

Causes of native-valve endocarditis
Streptococci
Viridans streptococci
Streptococcus bovis
Enterococci
Enterococcus faecalis
Enterococcus faecium
Staphylococcus aureus
Coagulase-negative staphylococci
Staphylococcus epidermidis
Staphylococcus lugdenensis
Streptococcus pneumoniae
HACEK group of organisms
Miscellaneous organisms
Culture-negative endocarditis

faecium) play an increasing role in endocarditis, particularly in the elderly and in those who have had invasive procedures in hospital. *Staphylococcus aureus* commonly attacks normal valves and presents very acutely with rapid valve destruction. Fungal infections and infection with Gram-negative bacteria are very rare.

ENDOCARDITIS IN INTRAVENOUS DRUG ABUSERS

The frequent use of nonsterile injection equipment predisposes intravenous drug abusers to endocarditis. In these patients, *S. aureus* is the most common pathogen. Fungal endocarditis is more common in abusers than in patients with native-valve endocarditis who are not abusers. In the past, infections by *Candida albicans* have resulted from contaminated lemon juice used to dissolve heroin before injection. Infections by pseudomonas also occur in this patient group. The majority of intravenous drug abusers develop endocarditis on previously normal valves; the tricuspid valve is the most commonly affected (**Fig. 5.2**), possibly because it is in direct line with the injected, contaminated drug. Involvement of the tricuspid valve frequently leads to septic emboli to the lungs.

PROSTHETIC VALVE ENDOCARDITIS

Modern cardiac surgery has led to an increase in valve replacement, usually with prosthetic material. Such material is more prone to infection and such infections are more difficult to eradicate than infections on native valves. In addition, blood flow through and around the prosthetic valves may be more turbulent, predisposing the valves to fibrin deposition and later infection.

Prosthetic valve endocarditis can be classed as 'early' or 'late'. Early prosthetic valve endocarditis appears within 60 days of valve implantation and usually results from perioperative infection; hence, staphylococci are the main culprits. Coagulase-negative staphylococci account for the majority of these infections (up to 30%), whereas *S. aureus* makes up about 20%. Late prosthetic valve endocarditis is more like native-valve endocarditis because the (abnormal) valve is covered by endothelium, so similar organisms occur in late prosthetic valve endocarditis as in native-valve endocarditis. However, staphylococci (both coagulase-negative and coagulase-positive types) play a more prominent role.

CULTURE-NEGATIVE ENDOCARDITIS

Some patients present with all the stigmata of endocarditis and may have vegetation on a valve, but blood cultures appear negative. Probably the most common cause of this is antibiotic therapy before blood culture. However, some fastidious organisms are difficult to culture (the HACEK group, **Fig. 5.3**) and prolonged cultures may be needed. Other

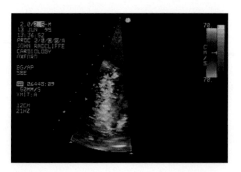

Fig. 5.2 *Echocardiogram showing tricuspid regurgitation.*

The HACEK organisms
Haemophilus aphrophilus *Actinobacillus actinomycetemcomitans* *Cardiobacterium hominis* *Eikenella corrodens* *Kingella kingae*

Fig. 5.3 *The HACEK group of organisms. Fastidious Gram-negative organisms causing endocarditis.*

organisms are extremely difficult or impossible to culture and their identification relies on serology or molecular techniques. These organisms are *Coxiella burnetii* (the cause of Q fever), chlamydia and bartonella.

PATHOLOGY

Endocarditis requires the presence of some form of damage to the heart valve in combination with the presence of organisms, usually bacteria, that adhere to the damaged valve. Valve damage may be caused by abnormal haemodynamics in the vicinity of the valve. High-pressure jets of blood passing through narrowed valve orifices may lead to endothelial damage. Turbulence around prosthetic valves or floppy mitral valves may also lead to damage. In addition, valves may be injured by the presence of central venous lines, angiography catheters or pacemaker wires. The injured endothelial surface encourages the deposition of fibrin and clumps of platelets as small vegetations. These are then ideal settings for the adherence of bacteria that enter the bloodstream. Transient bacteraemia may be related to purulent gingivitis, soft-tissue infections, damaged gastrointestinal epithelium or may follow invasive medical procedures such as venous cannulation. The bacteria adhere to the platelet–fibrin clump and promote further deposition of these components, effectively making the bacteria less accessible to phagocytes and antibiotics.

The presence of infection on the heart valves produces local cardiac effects as well as more distant problems. In the heart, infection can lead to valve perforation and rupture of the chordae tendinae. Abscesses may form around the valve (ring abscesses). Infection can also involve the conducting tissue, leading to rhythm disturbances. Very large vegetations may act like ball valves and obstruct the valve orifice. In addition, vegetations may detach from the valve and cause embolism in distant sites such as the cerebral vessels, the kidneys or even to the coronary arteries. Persistent bacteraemia may activate the immune system and often leads to the formation and circulation of immune complexes, which may be deposited at sites that are clinically apparent.

CLINICAL MANIFESTATIONS

Endocarditis may present acutely with obvious sepsis or may have a more subacute presentation, particularly with indolent organisms. The main clinical features of endocarditis are shown in **Figure 5.4**. Symptoms usually start within 2 weeks of the initial bacteraemia. Endocarditis caused by *S. aureus* often has a very acute onset. Although fever is the most common clinical finding in endocarditis, it should be noted that it is not always present.

Heart murmurs are usually audible. There may be a new murmur, or a previous murmur may change in character. A very acute onset of endocarditis in a person with normal valves may not be associated with any murmur. This is a not uncommon feature of acute endocarditis caused by *S. aureus*. Valve destruction or dysfunction often leads to cardiac failure, with symptoms and signs somewhat dependent on the affected valve. Cardiac failure may be more marked in those patients with pre-existing ischaemic heart disease. Infection involving the conducting tissue may cause arrhythmias, which may lead to worsening heart failure.

Embolic phenomena are common in endocarditis. They may be relatively minor, leading to splinter haemorrhages in the nail beds (**Fig. 5.5**), Janeway's lesions on the palms and soles (**Fig. 5.6**) or small renal infarcts leading to microscopic haematuria. Major emboli may lead to serious tissue damage. Cerebral vessels may be occluded, leading to strokes (**Fig. 5.7**). Renal and splenic abscesses can occur (**Fig. 5.8**), and septic lung emboli may be seen, particularly in tricuspid endocarditis. Immune complexes may cause glomerulonephritis, arthralgia and arthritis, and Osler's nodes. Osler's nodes are tender nodules (unlike Janeway's lesions) that occur on the pulps of the fingers and toes. Other features, such as splenomegaly and clubbing (**Fig. 5.9**), are rare nowadays and are only seen when the infection has been present and untreated for more than at least 6 weeks.

Clinical features of endocarditis

Symptoms	Signs
Fever	Fever
Rigors	Heart murmur
Dyspnoea	Changing or new murmur
Malaise	Embolic phenomena
Anorexia	Splinter haemorrhages
Weight loss	Splenomegaly
Back pain	Haematuria

Fig. 5.4 *Main clinical features of endocarditis.*

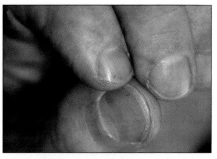

Fig. 5.5 *Splinter haemorrhages in a man with endocarditis affecting a ventriculoseptal defect.*

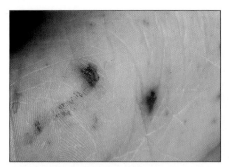

Fig. 5.6 *Feet showing numerous emboli in a man with endocarditis caused by* Staphylococcus aureus.

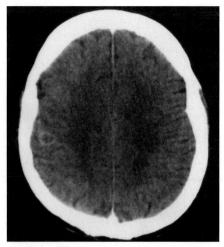

Fig. 5.7 *CT scan showing small abscesses in endocarditis caused by* Staphylococcus aureus

DIAGNOSIS

The mainstay of diagnosis is the demonstration in blood cultures of a persistent bacteraemia. Three sets of cultures should be taken at different times and anatomic sites over a 3–6 hour period and these will be positive in 95% of cases. Previous antibiotic therapy is the most common cause of negative cultures. Some organisms are particularly slow growing, so cultures should be incubated for at least 3 weeks before being discarded. Newer blood-culture systems allow earlier detection of organisms in the HACEK group. Endocarditis caused by *Coxiella burnettii* (Q fever) can only be diagnosed serologically or by molecular techniques such as polymerase chain reaction.

In addition to the clinical features already mentioned, echocardiography is an important adjunct to diagnosis. Transthoracic two-dimensional echocardiography can detect valvular dysfunction and vegetation (**Fig. 5.10**), but this technique has only a 50% sensitivity for vegetations. Alternatively, transoesophageal echocardiography (**Fig. 5.11**) increases the sensitivity for detecting vegetations to about 90% in experienced hands. Both techniques are operator dependent and a negative result cannot exclude endocarditis.

TREATMENT

Antibiotics

The choice of antibiotic therapy for endocarditis will depend on the organism isolated and its in-vitro sensitivities. Details are outlined in **Figure 5.12**, but some principles apply to all cases. The antibiotic should be bactericidal and should achieve good serum levels. This usually

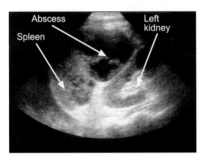

Fig. 5.8 *Ultrasonography of spleen shows large abscesses in endocarditis.*

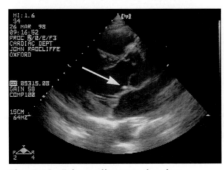

Fig. 5.10 *Echocardiogram showing vegetation on aortic valve.*

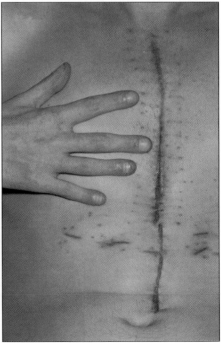

Fig. 5.9 *Clubbing is rare in endocarditis; this intravenous drug abuser had symptoms for more than 6 weeks.*

41

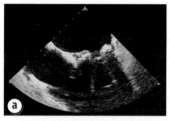 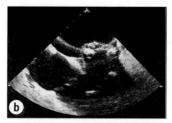

Fig. 5.11 *(a)* **Staphylococcus aureus** *infection of prosthetic mitral valve showing vegetation. (b) The infection has caused almost complete loosening of the valve so that it has changed its position during systole.*

Outline of antibiotic treatment of endocarditis

Streptococcal endocarditis
Benzylpenicillin 1.2g every 4 hours for 4 weeks
Benzylpenicillin (as above) plus gentamicin 80mg daily for 2 weeks
Benzylpenicillin and gentamicin (as above) but continue benzylpenicillin for a further
    2 weeks if organism is relatively penicillin resistant (minimal inhibitory concentration
    >0.1µg/ml)
Vancomycin 15mg/kg every 12 hours for 4 weeks

Enterococcal endocarditis
Ampicillin 2g every 4 hours plus gentamicin 1mg/kg every 8 hours for 4–6 weeks
Benzylpenicillin 2.4g every 4 hours plus gentamicin (as above) daily for 4–6 weeks
Vancomycin 15mg/kg every 12 hours plus gentamicin (as above) for penicillin-resistant
    enterococci (e.g. *Enterococcus faecium*)

Staphylococcus aureus endocarditis
Flucloxacillin or nafcillin 2g every 4 hours for 4–6 weeks
Above plus gentamicin 1mg/kg every 8 hours for 5 days
Vancomycin 15mg/kg every 12 hours for 4–6 weeks

Coagulase-negative staphylococcal endocarditis or methicillin-resistant *Staphylococcus aureus* endocarditis
Vancomycin 15mg/kg every 12 hours plus oral rifampicin 450mg every 12 hours
Vancomycin 15mg/kg every 12 hours plus gentamicin 1mg/kg every 8 hours

HACEK organisms
Ampicillin 2g every 4 hours plus gentamicin 1mg/kg every 8 hours for 4–6 weeks

Notes
1. Vancomycin regimens should be used in penicillin-allergic patients.
2. All drugs are give intravenously unless otherwise stated.
3. Gentamicin levels should be regularly monitored and the dosage adjusted accordingly.

Fig 5.12 *Antibiotic treatment of infectious endocarditis.*

requires high-dose intravenous therapy over a period of 4–6 weeks, although uncomplicated streptococcal endocarditis may be cured with 2 weeks' therapy. The patient must be closely monitored to ensure that the bacteraemia clears, clinical improvement occurs (such as the abatement of fever), no antibiotic toxicity is seen, and complications do not arise.

Persistence of fever usually implies a focus of infection (**Fig. 5.13**), most commonly a perivalvular abscess. Other foci include renal or splenic abscesses. Sometimes the antibiotics themselves may cause a fever; this may be accompanied by the formation and accumulation of an abnormally large number of eosinophils in the blood (eosinophilia).

Surgery

Cardiac surgery and valve replacement play an important role in the management of infectious endocarditis. Some generally accepted criteria for surgery are listed in **Fig. 5.14**. Valve replacement may be required for mechanical reasons, such as worsening heart failure caused by mitral regurgitation. Surgery may also be needed to eliminate foci of infection in the conducting system or to drain ring abscesses. Sometimes removal of an infected valve is the only way to control systemic sepsis, as is often the case with endocarditis caused by *S. aureus* (**Figs 5.15** and **5.16**). This condition usually requires surgery.

PROPHYLAXIS AGAINST ENDOCARDITIS

Spontaneous bacteraemia occurs from time to time in many people and is probably the most common cause of endocarditis. However, some dental and medical procedures are more likely to be associated with bacteraemia and, therefore, present a risk to those with abnormal heart valves. Although there is no definitive proof, interventions that traumatize

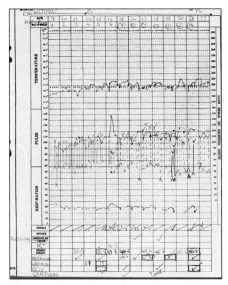

Fig 5.13 *Fever chart of a patient with splenic abscess after valve replacement.*

Criteria for surgery in endocarditis

Progressive heart failure
(caused by aortic valve regurgitation or rupture, or by rupture of chordae tendinae)
Persistent bacteraemia despite therapy
(may be caused by valve ring abscess or difficult-to-treat organisms)
Relapse after second course of antibiotics
Extension of infection into conducting system or pericardium

Fig 5.14 *Criteria for surgery in endocarditis.*

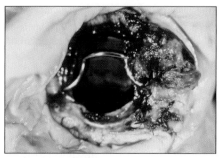

Fig 5.15 *Vegetations on prosthetic valve.*

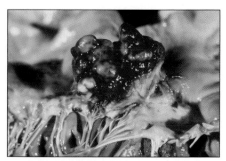

Fig 5.16 *Vegetations on mitral valve.*

Guidelines for antimicrobial prophylaxis against endocarditis

Types of patients
> Congenital heart disease (except simple atrial septal defect)
> Valvular heart disease
> Mitral valve prolapse (if systolic murmur present)
> Prosthetic heart valve
> Previously treated endocarditis
> Hypertrophic cardiomyopathy

Types of procedure
Dental extractions or scaling
> Amoxycillin 3g orally 1 hour before procedure
> * Clindamycin 600mg orally 1 hour before procedure
> * Erythromycin 1.5g orally 1 hour before procedure
> † Amoxycillin 1g intramuscularly and 0.5g orally 6 hours later
> †† Vancomycin 1g intravenously

Genitourinary or gastrointestinal tract manipulation [N.B. only required for those with prosthetic valves or a past history of endocarditis]
> Amoxycillin 1g intramuscularly and gentamicin 120mg intramuscularly and amoxycillin 0.5g intramuscularly (or orally) 6 hours later
> ‡ Vancomycin 1g intravenously and gentamicin 120mg intravenously or intramuscularly (option to repeat 12 hours later)

* alternative for penicillin-allergic subjects
† used if oral route is not available (i.e. procedure done under general anaesthetic)
‡ use if subject has had penicillin in past month or if penicillin allergic

Fig 5.17 *Guidelines for prophylaxis against endocarditis.*

the oral cavity, such as tooth extraction, are thought to carry a significant risk of endocarditis in susceptible individuals. Prophylaxis is directed against viridans streptococci (**Fig. 5.17**). For procedures that are likely to cause trauma to the genitourinary tract or the lower gastrointestinal tract, prophylaxis is directed against enterococci. Minor procedures, such as endoscopy or barium enema, only require prophylaxis if the patient has a prosthetic valve.

MYOCARDITIS

Inflammation of, and damage to, the heart muscle may be part of a systemic infection or may result from direct involvement of the heart. Myocarditis impairs myocardial contractility and hence reduces cardiac output (**Fig. 5.18**). Inflammation may also affect the cardiac conduction system (**Fig. 5.19**). The most common manifestations of myocarditis are, therefore, cardiac failure and arrhythmias. In practice, many patients with myocarditis also have pericarditis. The cause of infectious myocarditis is often not found, although viruses are the most common agents detected in cases in Europe and North America.

VIRAL MYOCARDITIS

Virus infections account for most cases of myocarditis. Enteroviruses (coxsackieviruses A and B, echoviruses, and polioviruses) are the most common pathogens to directly involve the myocardium. Often the infection is relatively benign with mild inflammation of the myocardium and moderate and transient impairment of cardiac function. Even in this setting, cardiac arrhythmias can occur, some fatal. Some infections have a much more aggressive course with marked inflammation and myocardial cell necrosis. This may rapidly progress to acute heart failure or fatal rhythm disturbance. Alternatively, progressive damage occurs, leading to a chronic cardiomyopathy, which may be either dilated or hypertrophic.

BACTERIAL MYOCARDITIS

About 10% of patients with Lyme disease may have cardiac involvement, usually affecting the conducting system. Legionella, mycoplasma and chlamydia may also produce myocarditis.

Myocarditis may be seen (but is relatively rare) in endocarditis caused by *S. aureus*, with the bacteria invading heart muscle and causing myocardial abscesses. Usually, pyogenic infections predominantly involve the pericardium with only slight involvement of the myocardium.

FUNGAL MYOCARDITIS

The myocardium may be invaded by fungi in systemic fungal infections, usually in immunocompromised hosts such as those receiving anticancer chemotherapy. Candida and aspergillus are the most common pathogens and frequently cause fungal abscesses in the myocardium.

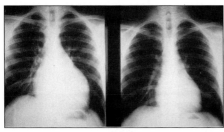

Fig 5.18 *Chest radiograph showing dilated heart in myocarditis (left); and after recovery (right).*

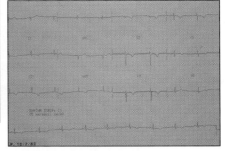

Fig. 5.19 *Electrocardiogram in myocarditis.*

PARASITES

In South America, infection with *Trypansoma cruzi* (Chagas' disease) leads to a cardiomyopathy. Toxoplasmosis can also cause a myocarditis, but usually only in immunosuppressed patients, especially heart-transplant recipients.

DIAGNOSIS

Clinical features include fever and evidence of cardiac dysfunction, such as cardiac failure or arrhythmias. The chest X-ray may show a large heart and the electrocardiogram may show arrhythmias or abnormal S–T segments. Echocardiography often shows global hypokinesia and this investigation should be performed serially to assess prognosis. Nuclear medicine scans, such as those using metastable technetium ($^{99}Tc^m$), may also help to assess function.

An etiologic diagnosis can be very difficult to prove. Endomyocardial biopsy may show acute or chronic inflammation (**Fig. 5.20**). This tissue may be cultured with traditional virologic techniques in an attempt to isolate the virus. Increasingly, molecular techniques to identify the presence of virus are proving useful. The isolation of a virus from noncardiac sites, such as the throat or from stool, is circumstantial evidence that the cardiac problem was caused by the virus. Less definitive diagnostic tests, that are rarely helpful diagnostically, include demonstrating a four-fold rise in antibodies to the specific virus on separate serum specimens or a single large antibody titre.

MANAGEMENT

In patients with myocarditis, the outcome is variable and depends on the infecting organism as well as on whether the patient has any pre-existing heart disease, such as coronary artery disease. Most treatment is symptomatic, aimed at controlling heart failure and arrhythmias. Because of the inflammation seen on myocardial biopsy specimens, anti-inflammatory drugs and immunosuppressive agents have been advocated for myocarditis. Recent studies have found no benefit with immunosuppression. With severe or chronic myocarditis, cardiac transplant may be required.

PERICARDITIS

Pericarditis may occur alone or in association with myocarditis. The same sort of organisms that cause myocarditis account for most cases of pericarditis, with enteroviruses as the leading cause. Pyogenic pericarditis is more common than pyogenic myocarditis. Fungal pericarditis usually occurs only in the immunosuppressed patient, but *Histoplasma capsulatum* may cause disease in immunocompetent patients in endemic areas.

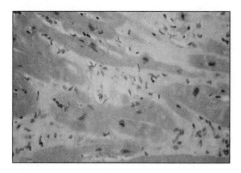

Fig. 5.20 *A cross-section showing inflammatory infiltrates in the myocardium (hematoxylin and eosin stain).*

CLINICAL MANIFESTATIONS

Patients with viral pericarditis are rarely very ill; the usual symptoms are malaise, fever and chest pain. On the other hand, those with bacterial pericarditis are toxic and ill. They are more prone to pericardial effusion and cardiac tamponade. Associated pleural effusions and ascites are also more common. Pericardial rubs can be heard in both viral and pyogenic cases but are not invariably present. Tuberculous pericarditis is chronic and most commonly is an incidental finding or later presents as constrictive pericarditis.

DIAGNOSIS

Pericarditis may be suspected clinically and confirmed by electrocardiography revealing widespread S–T changes, usually elevation (**Fig. 5.21**). Associated pericardial effusion may be suspected when a large, globular heart is seen on chest radiographs (**Fig. 5.22**) and low voltages are observed on electrocardiograms. Pericardial effusion is confirmed by echocardiography.

Wherever possible, pericardial fluid should be obtained for culture (viral, bacterial and fungal). Viral cultures of throat swabs and stool samples may detect enterovirus infections. The cause of the pericarditis can be inferred by changes in viral antibody titres in the serum, but this is not reliable. Pyogenic causes may be detected by blood culture or by culturing pericardial fluid. Tubercle bacilli are only cultured in about 40% of cases where pericardial fluid is examined, and pericardial biopsy may be useful in this condition (**Figs 5.23** and **5.24**).

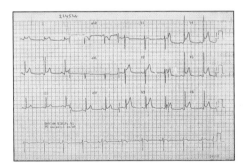

Fig. 5.21 *Electrocardiogram showing acute S–T changes in pericarditis.*

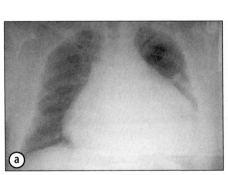

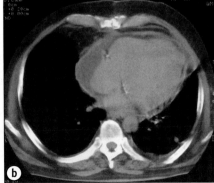

Fig. 5.22 *Staphylococcal pericarditis. (a) Chest radiograph showing huge cardiac shadow. (b) CT scan showing large collection of pus between pericardium and heart.*

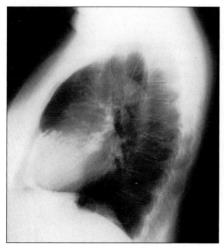

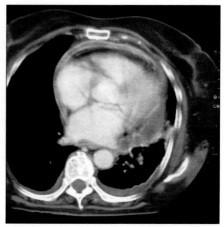

Fig. 5.23 *Calcified pericardium in tuberculous pericarditis.*

Fig. 5.24 *Computerized tomography shows thickened pericardium and pericardial effusion in tuberculous pericarditis.*

TREATMENT

Viral pericarditis can only be managed symptomatically. Pyogenic pericarditis, however, requires aggressive treatment. This means surgical pericardotomy and, usually, resection of the pericardium in addition to draining the purulent fluid. Parenteral antibiotics are required for at least 4 weeks. Tuberculous pericardial disease responds to appropriate antituberculous therapy. Steroids should be given in addition to antituberculous drugs to reduce the risk of subsequent constrictive pericarditis. Surgery is reserved for the few patients with tamponade or those who develop constriction.

ENDOVASCULAR INFECTIONS

Although the heart valves are the most common sites of infection in the circulation, infection can occur in vascular endothelium at other sites. This most commonly occurs at sites where there is endothelial damage secondary to atheromatous plaques, notably the abdominal aorta. Such plaques may become infected during bacteraemia (**Figs 5.25** and **5.26**). Although any organism may potentially cause endovascular infection, salmonella are well known to cause infection in native vessels, particularly in the elderly. In addition, septic emboli from endocarditic vegetations may give rise to infection elsewhere in the vascular tree, leading to so-called mycotic aneurysms. Any endovascular infection leads to vessel damage and carries the risk of aneurysm formation and rupture.

SEPTIC PHLEBITIS

Septic phlebitis may occur, either in association with indwelling central venous catheters or in intravenous drug users. Intravenous drug users may clinically exhibit obviously inflamed veins. Central venous catheters may become infected and this can present in a variety of ways. The exit site may become infected and infection can track up the subcutaneous tunnel, causing local cellulitis (**Fig. 5.27**). Infection of the line tip may result in bacteraemia;

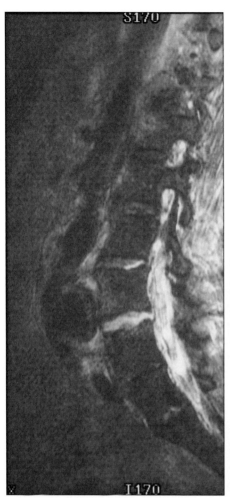

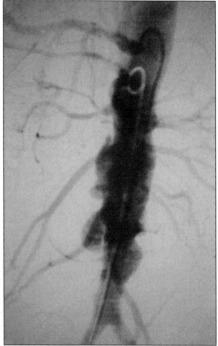

Fig. 5.26 *Angiographic image of mycotic aneurysm affecting the abdominal aorta.*

Fig. 5.25 *Magnetic resonance imaging shows mycotic aneurysm caused by Salmonella enteritidis with associated inflammation of the lumbar disc.*

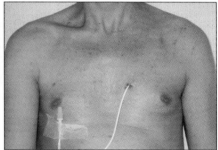

Fig. 5.27 *Tunnel infection involving a Hickman line. There is inflammation at the exit site and oedema in the supraclavicular fossa.*

if there is thrombus around the tip and along the vein, this may become infected. A variety of organisms may cause infection but the majority are coagulase-negative staphylococci, S. aureus and candida.

Tunnel infections and septic phlebitis require catheter removal and antibiotics. Bacteraemia caused by central venous lines may be treated with parenteral antibiotics without catheter removal. However, if the infective organism is *S. aureus* or a fungus, the line should come out.

INFECTION OF VASCULAR GRAFTS

The use of prosthetic material to replace aneurysmal vessels is now commonplace and these prosthetic vascular grafts can become infected. Such infections may occur at the time of surgery or later, following bacteraemia from another source (**Fig. 5.28**). The risk of vascular graft infection during surgery is increased if the operation is done as an emergency procedure, if repeat surgery is required (e.g. for postoperative bleeding), or if the groins are explored. The organisms involved are similar to those seen with prosthetic valve endocarditis, i.e. coagulase-negative staphylococci and *S. aureus*. However, anaerobes, enterobacteriacae, and enterococci also play a significant role in abdominal aortic graft infections because of the proximity of bowel (**Fig. 5.29**). Vascular graft infections may present with systemic symptoms of sepsis but more commonly present with local complications. False aneurysms, groin discharge, graft occlusion and distal emboli can all occur in femoro-popliteal graft infections (**Figs 5.30** and **5.31**). Abdominal aortic graft

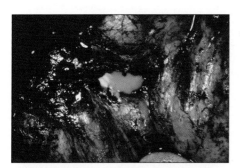

Fig. 5.28 *Perioperative view of pus around an aortic graft.*

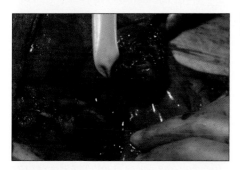

Fig. 5.29 *Aorto–duodenal fistula with bile staining of prosthetic graft.*

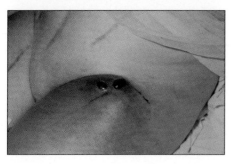

Fig. 5.30 *Acute infection of femoro-popliteal graft.*

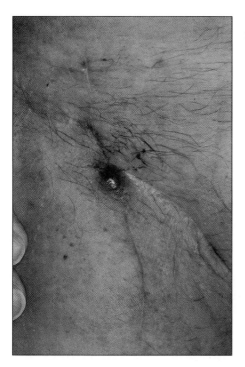

Fig. 5.31 *Chronic groin sinus with infected femoro-popliteal graft.*

infections may present with perigraft aneurysms, emboli, dehiscence or with upper gastrointestinal bleeding from an aorto–enteric fistula.

The management of endovascular infection is difficult. Mycotic aneurysms usually need surgical repair and prolonged antibiotic therapy. Vascular graft infections may need surgical treatment for local complications but the mainstay of treatment is intensive parenteral antibiotic therapy, followed by prolonged oral suppressive antibiotics.

chapter 6

Infections Involving the Respiratory Tract

This chapter deals with infective disorders of the upper and lower respiratory tracts and includes infections of the ears and oropharynx.

INFECTIONS OF THE ORAL CAVITY

CARIES

Caries is predominantly a disease of youth. It involves the demineralization of dental enamel. Tooth decay involves the action of acid that is produced from the fermentation of carbohydrates by bacteria in the mouth, notably *Streptococcus mutans* and, to a lesser extent, lactobacilli. Treatment has traditionally been mechanical with repair and restoration or removal of the affected teeth. Prevention is more important now and the role of fluoride is well established.

GINGIVITIS

Gingivitis may just be caused by local irritation, which may cause the gums to become reddened and slightly thicker than usual with a tendency to bleed after brushing the teeth. Acute infections, however, may lead to suppurative gingivitis (**Fig. 6.1**) or to acute necrotizing gingivitis (trench mouth).

In suppurative gingivitis there may be pus exuding from the gums with local pain. Systemic symptoms and signs of infection are more typical of acute necrotizing gingivitis and there is often accompanying halitosis and an abnormal taste. This is usually caused by anaerobes that are normally found in the oral cavity in addition to oral spirochaetes. Regional lymphadenopathy can occur. Acute necrotizing gingivitis often requires surgical debridement in addition to antibiotics such as metronidazole or tetracycline.

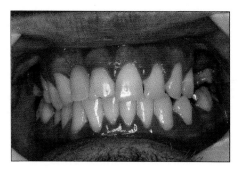

Fig. 6.1 *Severe gingivitis with redness and swelling of interdental papillae.*

DENTAL ABSCESSES

Dental abscess may occur if the dental pulp becomes infected, usually as a complication of caries. If untreated, the abscess may cause sufficient necrosis to go on to involve the alveolar bone (**Fig. 6.2**). Periodontal abscesses may occur around the apex of a tooth and often present as a focal inflammatory swelling in the gingivae.

MOUTH ULCERS

Ulceration of the oral mucosa may be caused by infection with either herpes simplex virus (HSV) or various types of enterovirus, usually Coxsackieviruses (**Fig. 6.3**). Diagnosis can be confirmed by isolation of the causative virus from ulcer swabs. Primary HSV infection is more commonly seen in children, in whom the inflammation and pain makes eating and drinking difficult (**Fig. 6.4**). Such patients may require intravenous fluids in addition to antiviral treatment. The hard palate may also be affected by varicella-zoster virus (VZV), either in chickenpox or in shingles affecting the maxillary division of the fifth cranial nerve (**Fig. 6.5**).

ACUTE EPIGLOTTITIS

Acute epiglottitis, which is usually caused by infection with *Haemophilus influenzae* type b, is likely to disappear in developed countries following the introduction of the *H. influenzae* type b conjugate vaccine. Acute epiglottitis occurs in children and usually causes a fever and dysphagia. The child often sits with its neck extended. Respiratory distress can occur because of partial airway obstruction; there is always the risk of acute obstruction and the need for tracheostomy (**Fig. 6.6**). Because of this risk, patients should be nursed in intensive

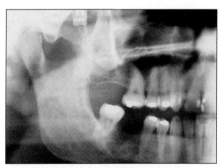

Fig. 6.2 *Osteomyelitis of the right mandible, following apical abscess and removal of the lower first molar.*

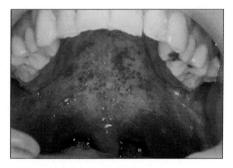

Fig. 6.3 *Vesicles on palate due to Coxsackievirus.*

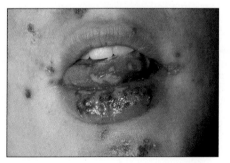

Fig. 6.4 *Primary herpes simplex virus (HSV) stomatitis.*

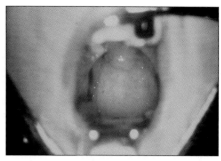

Fig. 6.6 *Acutely swollen epiglottis due to Haemophilus influenzae type b infection.*

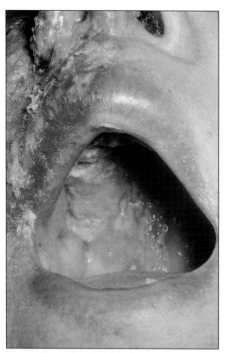

Fig. 6.5 *Herpes zoster of the maxillary division of the fifth cranial nerve.*

care and elective intubation may be indicated. Treatment with cefotaxime or chloramphenicol should be started once the diagnosis is suspected. Attempts to examine the airway or take swabs may provoke obstruction.

PHARYNGITIS

Most cases of acute pharyngitis are caused by viruses (**Fig. 6.7**) and, like most respiratory infections, this condition is more common in the winter. Some causes of pharyngitis, such as Epstein–Barr virus, lead to more severe sore throats than others, often with systemic symptoms. Bacterial sore throats are less common and are usually caused by group A β-haemolytic streptococci. Other streptococci, notably groups B and C, corynebacteria and anaerobes may also cause pharyngitis.

Glandular fever

Glandular fever (infectious mononucleosis) is caused by the Epstein–Barr virus. It leads to severe pharyngitis with tonsillar exudate in more than half of those infected (**Fig. 6.8**). Tonsillar enlargement may be so great that patients are unable to swallow anything, even their own saliva. Other features include fever, cervical lymphadenopathy and, frequently, splenomegaly. Atypical lymphocytes are seen in the blood film (**Fig. 6.9**) and the Paul–Bunnell heterophile antibody test is usually positive. If patients with acute Epstein–Barr virus infection are given ampicillin or amoxicillin they develop a florid erythematous, macular rash (**Fig. 6.10**). The rash eventually settles and does not signify penicillin allergy.

Causes of Pharyngitis

Viruses	Bacteria
Rhinovirus	Group A streptococci
Coronavirus	Other streptococci (groups B, C and G)
Adenovirus	*Corynebacterium diphtheriae*
Influenza virus A and B	Oro-pharyngeal anaerobes
Parainfluenza virus	*Neisseria gonorrhoeae*
Coxsackie A	*Treponema pallidum*
Herpes simplex virus (HSV)	*Arcanobacterium haemolyticum*
Epstein-Barr virus	
Cytomegalovirus	
HIV	

Fig. 6.7 *Causes of pharyngitis.*

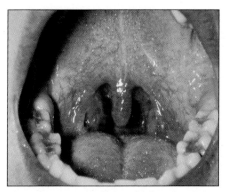

Fig. 6.8 *Pharyngitis due to Epstein–Barr virus.*

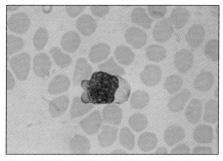

Fig. 6.9 *Blood film showing atypical monocyte in glandular fever.*

Fig. 6.10 *Ampicillin rash in patient with glandular fever.*

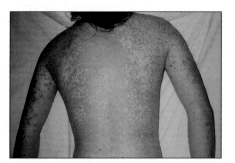

   Cytomegalovirus infection may also cause a mononucleosis-like syndrome but with much less marked pharyngitis and a negative Paul–Bunnell test. Primary human immunodeficiency virus (HIV) infection may lead to a similar illness, without tonsillar exudate, often in association with a maculopapular rash.

Streptococcal pharyngitis

Streptococcal pharyngitis, due to *Streptococcus pyogenes* infection, can range from mild to very severe and can be clinically identical to the pharyngitis of glandular fever (**Fig. 6.11**). There is usually a fever and raised white cell count. Toxin production from some strains of group A streptococci may lead to scarlet fever or to toxic shock syndrome.

Scarlet fever is characterized by an erythematous rash (**Fig. 6.12**), which subsequently desquamates, and a bright red 'strawberry' tongue (**Fig. 6.13**).

DIPHTHERIA

Infection with *Corynebacterium diphtheriae*, and sometimes with *Corynebacterium ulcerans*, produces respiratory symptoms and pharyngitis in the first week of illness. The disease is characterized by a low-grade fever and the formation of a white–grey pharyngeal membrane that extends, initially, from the tonsils to cover the soft palate and uvula (**Fig. 6.14**). The membrane is often markedly adherent to the mucosa, and attempts at

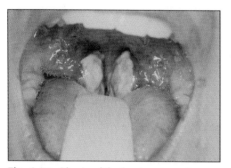

Fig. 6.11 *Pharyngitis due to group A streptococcal infection.*

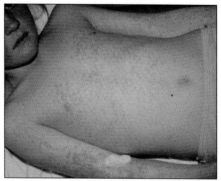

Fig. 6.12 *Scarletina rash in scarlet fever.*

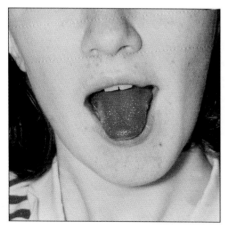

Fig. 6.13 *'Strawberry' tongue in scarlet fever.*

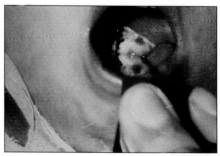

Fig. 6.14 *Grey tonsillar membrane in acute diphtheria.*

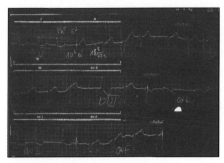

Fig. 6.15 *Complete heart block in diphtheria.*

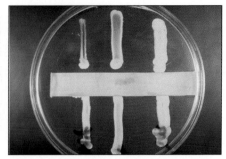

Fig. 6.16 *Elek plate demonstrating toxin from* Corynebacterium diphtheriae.

removing it may cause bleeding. In severe cases, the membrane may advance sufficiently to cause respiratory obstruction, a not uncommon feature in the prevaccination era. Nasal diphtheria, when the nasal mucosa is involved by membrane, may present with purulent and sometimes serosanguinous nasal discharge.

During the second week of illness, diphtheria toxin may cause a myocarditis with a variety of conduction defects (**Fig. 6.15**) and cardiac dilatation. Cardiac failure and cardiac arrest may occur. In addition, a proportion of patients may get neurological symptoms, usually as a result of peripheral polyneuropathy, although sometimes the cranial nerves are involved.

Diphtheria is diagnosed clinically and by culture of the organism from throat swabs. Toxin production can be identified *in vitro* by the Elek test (**Fig. 6.16**). Treatment is with the combination of antibiotics (erythromycin or benzylpenicillin) and specific antitoxin. Immunization with diphtheria toxoid prevents the severe manifestations of the disease.

HEAD AND NECK SPACE INFECTIONS

Infection in the oropharynx may spread to the soft tissues of the head and neck, sometimes with serious consequences. These sorts of complications were much more common in the preantibiotic era but they still occasionally occur today.

PROBLEMS RELATING TO DENTAL SEPSIS

Masticator space infection
The muscles of mastication (the masseters, temporalis and pterygoids) have potential spaces around them that may become sites of abscesses. Such abscesses most commonly follow tooth infections, usually of the upper molars and especially of the 'wisdom' teeth. Such infections present with pain and trismus (inability to fully open the mouth).

Ludwig's angina
Ludwig's angina is a spreading cellulitis that affects the floor of the mouth, usually following dental abscess or extraction. It leads to a bilateral involvement of the sublingual and submandibular spaces and swollen, indurated tissue without abscess formation (**Fig. 6.17**).

INFECTIONS RELATING TO PHARYNGITIS
The soft tissues of the neck may be infected by contiguous spread from the pharynx and, rarely, as a complication of dental or ear infections.

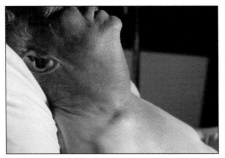

Fig. 6.17 *Swollen neck in Ludwig's angina.*

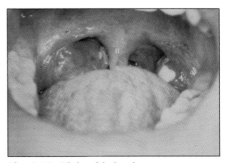

Fig. 6.18 *Right-sided quinsy, or peritonsillar abscess.*

Quinsy

The quinsy, or peritonsillar abscess, is an infrequent complication of bacterial tonsillitis. It presents as a very painful, unilateral swelling in one tonsillar bed (**Fig. 6.18**). There is usually a degree of trismus along with a fever and dysphagia. Intraoral drainage and antibiotics are required.

Parapharyngeal abscess

If untreated, peritonsillar abscesses may progress and involve the lateral pharyngeal spaces (**Fig. 6.19**). If the parapharyngeal abscess is located anteriorly, there may be trismus and dsyphagia with displacement of the pharyngeal wall and swelling of the parotid gland. Posterior infection may lead to respiratory obstruction if there is laryngeal oedema. There may also be cranial nerve involvement and there is a risk of invasion through to the carotid artery or jugular vein.

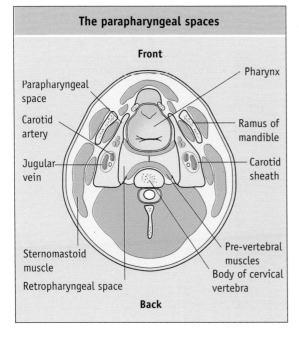

The parapharyngeal spaces

Front

Pharynx

Parapharyngeal space

Carotid artery

Ramus of mandible

Jugular vein

Carotid sheath

Sternomastoid muscle

Pre-vertebral muscles

Body of cervical vertebra

Retropharyngeal space

Back

Fig. 6.19 *The parapharyngeal spaces.*

Retropharyngeal abscess

Pharyngitis may spread backwards to the retropharyngeal lymph glands which then suppurate. These abscesses are more common in children because the glands atrophy with age. In children, and sometimes in adults, trauma to the pharynx by lollipop sticks or fish bones may lead to abscess formation. They may also be caused by the trauma of an upper gastrointestinal endoscopy. Children may have few localizing signs and may present simply with fever, lethargy and refusal to eat. Adults usually have pain, dysphagia and fever. There may be dysphonia and, sometimes, neck swelling, drooling of saliva and neck stiffness. This condition may be mistaken for meningitis or cervical osteomyelitis but a retropharyngeal abscess may be seen on a plain lateral radiograph of the neck (**Fig. 6.20**).

Treatment

These soft tissue infections (quinsy, parapharyngeal abscess and retropharyngeal abscess) of the neck are usually polymicrobial, reflecting the oropharyngeal flora. Successful treatment requires prompt diagnosis, appropriate intravenous antibiotics (including anaerobic cover) and surgical drainage. Complications include bleeding and respiratory obstruction. Particularly serious is posterior spread of infection to involve the carotid sheath, which contains both the carotid artery and the internal jugular vein. Erosion into the artery causes catastrophic haemorrhage and invasion of the jugular vein leads to a septic thrombophlebitis and consequent septic pulmonary emboli, with metastatic abscesses.

INFECTION OF THE SALIVARY GLANDS

Mumps used to be the most common cause of parotid and other salivary gland swelling. This disease, caused by a paramyxovirus, is now extremely uncommon in developed

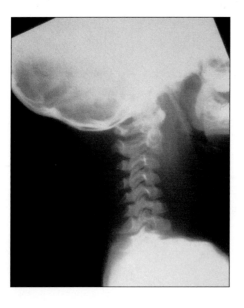

Fig. 6.20 *Lateral neck X-ray showing a retropharyngeal abscess.*

countries because of routine immunization against the virus. It usually presents with fever, malaise and bilateral parotid swelling (**Fig. 6.21**). Recognized complications include orchitis and pancreatitis, both of which are usually mild. Mumps used to be the most common cause of benign lymphocytic meningitis. Other viruses, such as influenza and enteroviruses, may cause parotitis, as may HIV.

Suppurative sialadenitis is often secondary to stones blocking either Stensen's duct (in the case of the submandibular glands) or Wharton's duct (in the case of the parotid glands). The former is more common. Suppurative parotitis may occur in the absence of stones in malnourished or debilitated patients. There is usually local pain and unilateral swelling with concomitant systemic features such as fever and rigors. *Staphylococcus aureus* is a common cause but Enterobacteraceae and anaerobes may be involved. Treatment requires antibiotics and surgical drainage.

EAR INFECTIONS

OTITIS EXTERNA

Superficial otitis externa
Otitis externa is usually a superficial infection of the external auditory canal. The condition often involves *Pseudomonas* spp. and is usually associated with moisture. There is erythema and exudate in the canal, often with oedema (**Fig. 6.22**). The ear-drum may be involved but it moves normally with pressure. For treatment, local antiseptic or antibiotic drops are usually adequate.

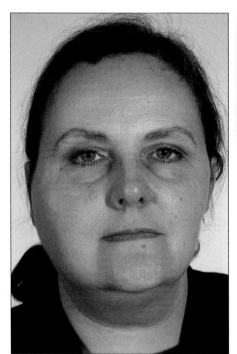

Fig. 6.21 *Mumps parotitis.*

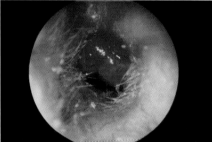

Fig. 6.22 *Inflamed external meatus in otitis externa.*

Malignant otitis externa

Malignant otitis externa is a serious infection that can involve deep soft tissue and bone. It is usually seen in elderly people with diabetes mellitus and is almost always caused by *Pseudomonas aeruginosa*. Patients complain of pain, redness and discharge. There may be marked cellulitis with local necrosis (**Fig. 6.23**). Aggressive antibiotic therapy with antipseudomonal β-lactam agents in combination with an aminoglycoside is required. Debridement may be needed if there is extensive bony involvement. In some cases a facial nerve palsy occurs.

OTITIS MEDIA

Otitis media is usually a disease of childhood. Acute suppurative otitis media is an acute infection of the middle ear that should be distinguished from chronic secretory otitis media, in which serous fluid accumulates in the middle ear. Acute otitis media is rare after the age of 5 years and usually presents with fever and pain following upper respiratory tract symptoms. There may be purulent discharge from the ear. Diagnosis can be difficult; classically the drum appears red and bulging (**Fig. 6.24**) and has no movement to pressure from a pneumatic otoscope.

Both bacterial and viral infections can lead to acute otitis media. *Streptococcus pneumoniae* and *H. influenzae* are the most common bacterial causes but mycoplasmas also play a role. Upper respiratory tract viruses have been implicated in up to a quarter of cases, with respiratory syncytial virus (RSV) being the most common.

Management usually involves giving antibiotics to cover *S. pneumoniae* and *H. influenzae*. The role of myringotomy is controversial. Untreated otitis media can, rarely, go on to invade the meninges, resulting in bacterial meningitis.

MASTOIDITIS

Chronic suppurative otitis media usually involves the mastoid and results from repeated or chronic pyogenic middle ear infections. Although the organisms causing acute otitis media may be found in this condition, more commonly Gram-negative bacteria (such as *Pseudomonas* spp.) and staphylococci are found. There is usually pain in the affected ear (**Fig. 6.25**) and there may be purulent discharge through a perforated ear-drum. Computed tomography (CT) scanning and magnetic resonance imaging (MRI) are useful for diagnosis and for excluding complications such as osteomyelitis and cholesteatoma.

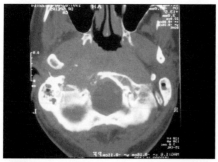

Fig. 6.23 *Malignant otitis externa caused by* Pseudomonas *spp., causing osteomyelitis of the base of the skull, seen on axial CT scan.*

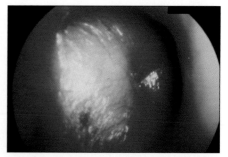

Fig. 6.24 *Bulging tympanic membrane in otitis media.*

SINUSITIS

Acute sinusitis

Acute sinusitis, like otitis media, can be caused by a variety of respiratory viruses and bacteria. In children, this may present just with a cough or a runny nose. Adults more frequently have headache and localized pain, and sometimes fever. Diagnosis may be helped by transillumination of the sinus or by plain X-ray (**Fig. 6.26**). However, CT and MRI scans are more sensitive and specific. Sinus puncture and, increasingly, sinus endoscopy (**Fig. 6.27**) enable microbiological specimens to be obtained and can be used therapeutically

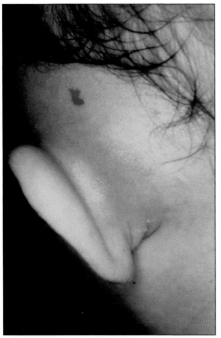

Fig. 6.25 *Acute mastoiditis: inflammation behind the ear.*

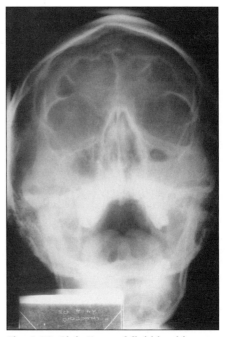

Fig. 6.26 *Plain X-ray of fluid level in maxillary sinus in acute sinusitis.*

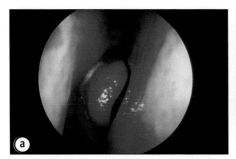
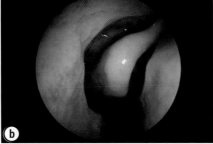

Fig. 6.27 *Acute sinusitis: (a) endoscopic view before treatment showing oedematous turbinates; (b) endoscopic view after treatment showing that the oedema has resolved.*

to drain infected secretions. Antibiotics active against the common respiratory bacterial pathogens should be used. Decongestants and antihistamines are often used in conjunction with antibiotics for sinusitis but their role has never been critically evaluated.

Chronic sinusitis

Chronic sinusitis may sometimes be due to chronic infection, although allergy and inflammatory polyps also play a significant role. For symptoms caused by chronic sepsis, antibiotics alone are rarely effective and usually need to be given in conjunction with some form of surgical drainage procedure.

BRONCHITIS

ACUTE BRONCHITIS

Acute bronchitis is usually viral in origin, although sometimes bacteria such as *Mycoplasma pneumoniae* or *Chlamydia pneumoniae* may be implicated. People with normal lungs can be affected and the condition resolves spontaneously. There is little evidence that antibiotic therapy affects outcome.

ACUTE BRONCHIOLITIS

Acute bronchiolitis is usually seen only in infants under the age of 2 years and is most common in the winter months. It is normally due to RSV (**Fig. 6.28**) although other viruses (**Fig. 6.29**) and occasionally *M. pneumoniae* may be the cause.

Symptoms usually begin with a cough and coryza and progress over a few days. Wheezing is common and bronchiolitis may therefore be confused with asthma. Bronchiolitis may lead to respiratory distress but usually resolves with symptomatic treatment.

PERTUSSIS

Pertussis, or whooping cough, is sometimes known as the one-hundred-days cough. Although the disease predominantly affects children, it may also occur in susceptible adults. *Bordetella pertussis* is the usual cause although *Bordetella parapertussis* may lead to the same syndrome.

The disease usually begins with cold-like symptoms before the cough develops. The cough becomes explosive and occurs in paroxysms. Such paroxysms may lead to apnoeic episodes in young children. The organism may be cultured from pernasal swabs or aspirates early in the course of the disease. Antibiotics shorten the disease only slightly but they do reduce infectivity. Immunization is the best means of preventing pertussis.

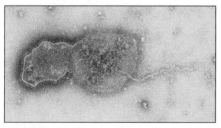

Fig. 6.28 *Electron micrograph of respiratory syncytial virus (RSV); partial disruption has occured releasing a strand of ribonucleic acid.*

Causes of bronchiolitis

Respiratory syncytial virus (RSV)
Parainfluenza virus (types 1 and 3)
Adenovirus
Influenza virus
Coronavirus
Rhinovirus
Measles virus
Mycoplasma pneumoniae

Fig. 6.29 *Causes of bronchiolitis.*

CHRONIC BRONCHITIS

The term 'chronic bronchitis' implies inflammation of an already damaged respiratory tract. This condition is often defined clinically as a productive cough for at least 3 consecutive months for more than 2 years in succession. Cigarette smoking, air pollution and inhaled dust are important aetiological factors but infections may lead to disease exacerbations. *S. pneumoniae*, *H. influenzae* and *Moraxella catarrhalis* are the bacteria most frequently associated with exacerbations of chronic bronchitis; viral pathogens can also be involved. For severe exacerbations, antibiotic therapy probably leads to earlier resolution of symptoms.

BRONCHIECTASIS

Bronchiectasis is a condition in which the airways are permanently dilated. It may arise from a variety of different insults to the lungs (**Fig. 6.30**). Although bronchiectasis is often generalized, it may be focal, as may occur distal to an obstructed bronchus. Cystic fibrosis is the most common cause of generalized bronchiectasis.

Clinical symptoms vary according to how much lung is involved in the disease process. Usually, there is a chronic cough with the production of large amounts of purulent sputum, sometimes with associated haemoptysis. Coarse crackles may be heard on auscultation and there may be wheezing. Finger clubbing is common. Bronchiectasis is now best confirmed by CT scan of the lungs (**Figs 6.31** and **6.32**).

Treatment is aimed at correcting any underlying reversible cause, providing physiotherapy, usually with postural drainage (**Fig. 6.33**), appropriate antibiotic treatment of infective flare-ups and, occasionally, surgery.

Causes of bronchiectasis		
Postinfective	**Host defects**	**Bronchial obstruction**
Measles pneumonia	Immunoglobulin deficiencies (primary and secondary)	Foreign body
		Tumour
Whooping cough	Chronic granulomatous disease	Lymph node
Mycoplasmal infections	Cystic fibrosis	
Adenoviruses	Kartagener's syndrome	
Tuberculosis	HIV infection	
α-1 antitrypsin deficiency	Yellow nail syndrome	

Fig. 6.30 *Causes of bronchiectasis.*

PNEUMONIA

VIRAL PNEUMONIA

Viral pneumonias are more common in children than adults. They may be caused by any of the viruses that lead to acute bronchitis. Measles pneumonia used to be common but is rarely seen in developed countries today. However, it is still a significant cause of morbidity and mortality in the tropics. Chickenpox pneumonia (**Figs 6.34** and **6.35**) can be very

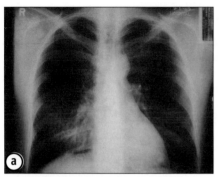

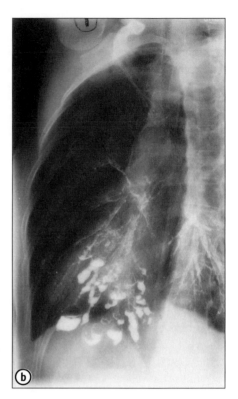

Fig. 6.31 *Bronchiectasis: (a) chest radiograph of basal bronchiectasis. (b) bronchogram showing dilated bronchi. (These investigations have now been superceded by CT scanning.)*

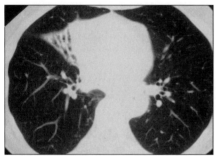

Fig. 6.32 *CT scan of bronchiectasis.*

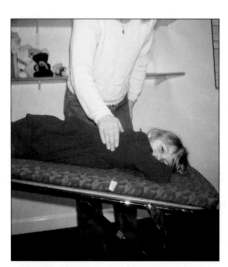

Fig. 6.33 *Patient with cystic fibrosis undergoing postural drainage.*

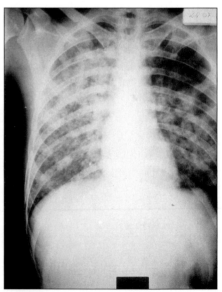

Fig. 6.34 *Pulmonary infiltrates in an adult with chickenpox.*

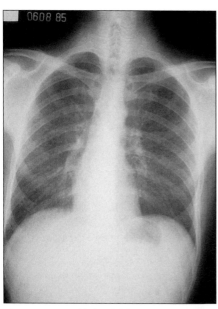

Fig. 6.35 *Speckled calcification in lungs after chickenpox pneumonitis.*

Organisms causing community acquired pneumonia*

Streptococcus pneumoniae
Influenza virus
Mycoplasma pneumoniae
Legionella pneumophila
Haemophilus influenzae
Chlamydia pneumoniae
Coxiella burnetii (Q fever)
Staphylococcus aureus
Various other viruses

* in up to a third of cases, no causative organism can be identified

Fig. 6.36 *Organisms causing community-acquired pneumonia. Note that in up to one-third of cases, no causative organism can be identified.*

severe in adults, sometimes causing death. Other herpes viruses usually cause pneumonia only in immunocompromised patients. Measles in children and influenza in adults may be complicated by the development of secondary bacterial pneumonia, often caused by *S. aureus*.

BACTERIAL PNEUMONIA

Community-acquired pneumonia

Community-acquired pneumonia usually occurs sporadically but there may be epidemics. Usually caused by pyogenic bacteria, other so-called atypical bacteria are increasingly recognized as causes of pneumonia (**Fig. 6.36**). Patients typically present with cough and fever, and they may be breathless or have pleuritic pain. Some patients, particularly if they are bacteraemic, may have systemic symptoms such as vomiting or diarrhoea or may be in septic shock. In addition to fever and tachypnoea, signs of consolidation may be present with coarse crackles and bronchial breathing on auscultation.

Pneumococcal pneumonia

Pneumococcal pneumonia (caused by *S. pneumoniae*) is the most common community acquired pneumonia and is the most likely to be associated with bacteraemia (30% of cases). Symptoms come on acutely, and clinical and radiographic signs of consolidation are common (**Fig. 6.37**). Some patients with immunosuppression may be more prone to infection with *S. pneumoniae* (e.g. those with HIV infection, hypogammaglobulinaemia or myeloma). Benzylpenicillin used to be the treatment of choice, but the spread of penicillin-resistant pneumococci is increasing and therefore, in some settings, third-generation cephalosporins or glycopeptides may be needed.

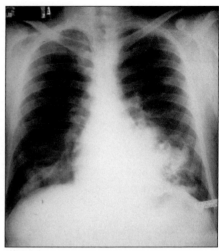

Fig. 6.38 *Multiple lung abscesses in* Staphylococcus aureus *pneumonia.*

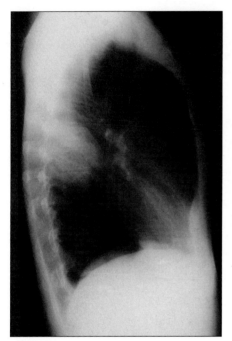

Fig. 6.37 *Lobar consolidation in pneumococcal pneumonia.*

Haemophilus influenzae pneumonia

H. influenzae, particularly encapsulated strains, may lead to pneumonia but such infection is more difficult to see on Gram stain. It is a less common cause of community-acquired pneumonia than the pneumococcus but is identical in clinical presentation.

Staphylococcal pneumonia

Staphylococcal pneumonia, due to *S. aureus* infection, may account for up to 10% of cases of community-acquired pneumonia. There may be patchy, bilateral consolidation on chest X-ray and, unlike the situation in most bacterial pneumonias, early abscess formation and cavitation is common (**Fig. 6.38**). Staphylococcal pneumonia occurs more frequently in elderly patients following influenza and is more common in intravenous drug users, when it may be a sign of *S. aureus* endocarditis of the tricuspid valve.

Klebsiella pneumoniae pneumonia

Klebsiella pneumoniae as a cause of community-acquired pneumonia is relatively rare but, like staphylococcal pneumonia, it may lead to early cavitation.

Legionnaires' disease

Legionnaires' disease, caused by *Legionella pneumophila*, is an example of a so-called 'atypical pneumonia'. It is more common in men and in those who smoke. In the UK it is also recognized as being more common as a cause of pneumonia in returning travellers. Patients with legionnaires' disease may be very ill and require intensive care treatment but, in general, there are no clinical features that reliably differentiate infections with *Legionella* spp. from other bacterial pneumonias (**Fig. 6.39**).

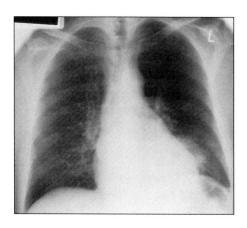

Fig. 6.39 *Bilateral pneumonia in legionnaires' disease.*

Mycoplasma pneumoniae pneumonia

Mycoplasma pneumoniae is responsible for pneumonia occurring in previously healthy people, particularly young adults. In the UK, epidemics of this infection occur in 4-yearly cycles. The pneumonia is usually mild and self-limiting but it responds to macrolides (e.g. erythromycin) or tetracyclines.

Chlamydial pneumonia

Chlamydia pneumoniae, formerly known as TWAR, is increasingly recognized as a cause of community-acquired pneumonia. Its clinical manifestations are indistinguishable from those of other causes of pneumonia. Less frequently, *Chlamydia psittaci*, may cause pneumonia; some cases are associated with exposure to birds.

Q fever

Q fever, caused by the rickettsia *Coxiella burnetii* may present as a pneumonia. Because this organism is associated with cattle, farm workers and veterinary surgeons may be at increased risk.

Nosocomial pneumonia

Nosocomial pneumonia, or pneumonia acquired in hospital, may occur postoperatively or may be seen in the intensive care setting in intubated, ventilated patients (Fig. 6.40). Nosocomial infections also occur in patients who are immunocompromised as a result of therapy or disease (see Chapter 13). Although the same sort of organisms that cause

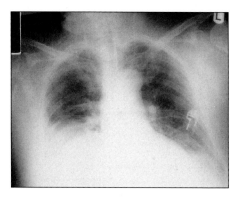

Fig. 6.40 *Ventilator-associated pneumonia.*

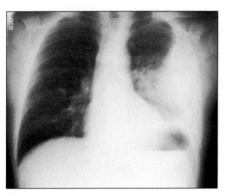

Fig. 6.41 *Pleural empyema with pneumococcal pneumonia.*

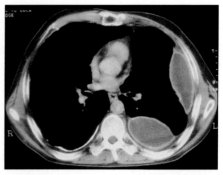

Fig. 6.42 *CT scan of the chest showing empyema.*

Fig. 6.43 *Chest drain to treat empyema.*

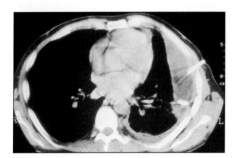

community-acquired pneumonias may be involved in nosocomial infections, the usual pathogens are Gram-negative bacteria, such as the Enterobacteriaceae (e.g. *E. coli*) and *Pseudomonas* spp.

EMPYEMA

Pleural effusions are often present in acute pneumonia but when these become infected and purulent, an empyema occurs. These often become loculated and act as an intrathoracic abscess (**Figs 6.41** and **6.42**), causing local pain and swinging fevers. In addition to antibiotic treatment, the empyema needs to be drained, either percutaneously (**Figs 6.43** and **6.44**) or by an open surgical procedure. Trials are currently underway to determine if the percutaneous instillation of thrombolytic agents aids drainage and hastens resolution of empyemas. Increasingly, thoracoscopy is being used to investigate the cause of pleural effusions (**Figs 6.45** and **6.46**).

LUNG ABSCESSES

Lung abscesses can either form as a result of aspiration or as a consequence of haematogenous spread of bacteria to the lung. Aspiration may occur during periods of

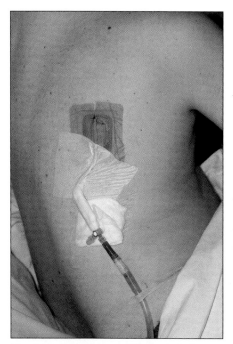

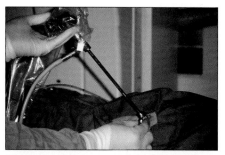

Fig. 6.45 *Thorasoscopy being performed.*

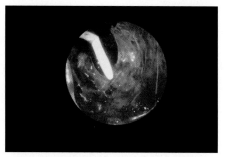

Fig. 6.44 *Chest X-ray with chest drain to treat empyema.*

Fig. 6.46 *Thoracoscopic view of empyema showing fibrin adhesions which are responsible for the loculation of pus commonly encountered.*

unconsciousness, e.g. in alcoholic or diabetic coma (**Fig. 6.47**) or following a generalized seizure, and it may lead to a single lung abscess, usually in the right lung. The bacteria involved in abscess formation in such circumstances are usually oropharyngeal aerobic and anaerobic organisms, which are almost invariably susceptible to penicillin. Bacteraemia with organisms such as *S. aureus* or the *Streptococcus milleri* group may lead to multiple lung abscesses (**Fig. 6.48**).

ASPERGILLUS INFECTIONS

A variety of fungi may infect the lungs, usually in immunocompromised patients. The most common species to do so is *Aspergillus*. This fungus may involve the lungs in a variety of ways.

ALLERGIC BRONCHOPULMONARY ASPERGILLOSIS

This condition occurs in patients with known asthma. It presents with breathlessness, a peripheral blood eosinophilia and fleeting pulmonary infiltrates on chest X-ray. Patients have a hypersensitivity to *Aspergillus* antigen, which can be shown on skin testing. The bronchi become intermittently plugged with aspergilli, which are usually found in the sputum. Symptoms frequently resolve with steroids and the fungus does not become invasive. However, some patients may develop bronchiectasis or poorly controlled, steroid-dependent asthma.

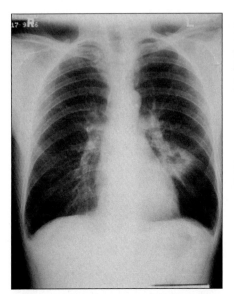

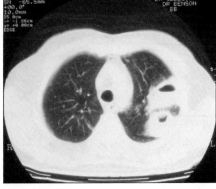

Fig. 6.48 *CT scan showing lung abscesses caused by* Streptococcus milleri.

Fig. 6.47 *Lung abscess on plain X-ray in a diabetic following hypoglycaemic coma.*

ASPERGILLOMA

Patients with pre-existing lung cavities, such as those from previous tuberculosis or from bronchiectasis, may develop fungal balls within the cavities after inhaling the fungal spores and becoming colonized (**Fig. 6.49**). These patients may be at risk from haemorrhage from the involved cavity. They usually have markedly raised IgG antibodies to *Aspergillus* in the serum and intermittently have the fungus in their sputum.

INVASIVE ASPERGILLOSIS

This is a serious complication of immunocompromised patients, particularly those with neutropenia. Pulmonary infiltrates and fever occur (**Fig. 6.50**). The fungal hyphae invade through the lung and may involve blood vessels, leading either to haemorrhage or to metastatic infection, commonly in the brain. This condition carries a high mortality even in the face of appropriate therapy.

TUBERCULOSIS

Pulmonary disease accounts for about 80% of all disease resulting from infection with *Mycobacterium tuberculosis*. Most *M. tuberculosis* infections are acquired by the respiratory route. The infecting organisms pass from the lung parenchyma to local, usually hilar, lymph nodes and from there can disseminate via the bloodstream. In immunocompetent persons, dissemination is stopped by the development of cell-mediated immunity within 1 month to 6 weeks of infection. Organisms may be contained rather than eliminated, posing a risk of later reactivation.

PRIMARY INFECTION

Most primary infections are asymptomatic but some children and a few adults have fever, cough and shortness of breath. There may be signs of consolidation in the chest and the

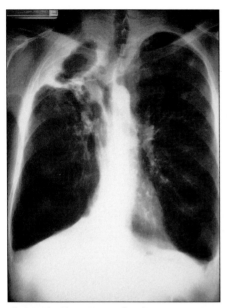

Fig. 6.49 *Chest X-ray showing aspergilloma in an old tuberculosis cavity.*

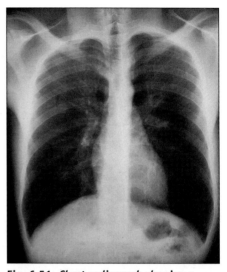

Fig. 6.51 *Chest radiograph showing a primary complex in tuberculosis; hilar lymphadenopathy with ipsilateral consolidation.*

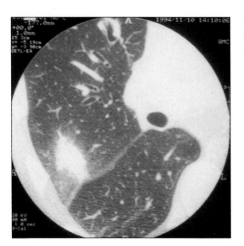

Fig. 6.50 *CT scan showing invasive aspergillosis in a patient with acute myeloid leukaemia.*

chest X-ray may show a primary complex – an area of consolidation in the lower part of an upper lobe or in the upper parts of the middle or lower lobes, in association with ipsilateral hilar (or sometimes paratracheal) lymph node enlargement (**Fig. 6.51**). Some patients may develop an allergic reaction to *M. tuberculosis* with primary infection. This may take the form of erythema nodosum, a reactive polyarthritis (Poncet's disease) or phlyctenular conjunctivitis. About 10% of cases of primary *M. tuberculosis* infection go on within a few months to develop symptomatic pulmonary tuberculosis. A few patients, particularly children, may get severe disseminated disease, or miliary tuberculosis.

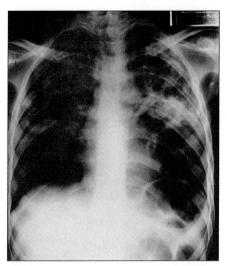

Fig. 6.52 *Typical chest X-ray of pulmonary tuberculosis.*

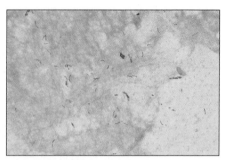

Fig. 6.53 *Sputum stained with Ziehl–Neelsen stain showing acid-fast bacilli.*

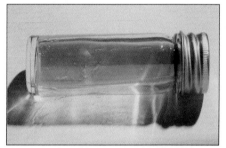

Fig. 6.54 *Lowenstein–Jensen medium with colonies of* Mycobacterium tuberculosis.

PULMONARY TUBERCULOSIS

Patients with pulmonary tuberculosis may present with a variety of symptoms; about 20% will be relatively asymptomatic despite an abnormal chest X-ray (**Fig. 6.52**). Most patients develop a cough and have some malaise and weight loss. Only about half have a persistent fever and a quarter develop haemoptysis. The disease is characterized by caseating granulomas and is often locally destructive, leading to the formation of cavities. Cavitating disease is highly infectious.

Diagnosis is made by the finding of acid-fast bacilli in the sputum (**Fig. 6.53**) and positive sputum culture for *M. tuberculosis* (**Fig. 6.54**). If sputum is not being produced, samples may be obtained by induced sputum procedures or by obtaining early morning gastric aspirate (to recover acid-fast bacilli from respiratory secretions that have been swallowed). The best yields are from bronchoalveolar lavage. Patients who are sputum-positive on microscopy should be isolated in a single room for the first 2 weeks of treatment.

Pulmonary tuberculosis may be complicated by massive haemoptysis if cavities erode major vessels. Enlarging lymph nodes may compress adjacent bronchi, causing secondary infection and bronchiectasis. Occasionally, cavities may be secondarily infected with *Aspergillus* spp., leading to an aspergilloma.

TUBERCULOUS PLEURISY

When subpleural caseaseous plaques rupture into the pleural space, the resulting inflammation leads to the formation of an effusion (**Fig. 6.55**). This may follow primary

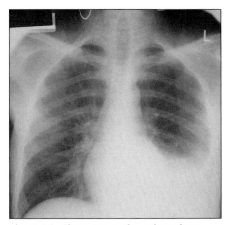

Fig. 6.55 *Chest X-ray of a tuberculous pleural effusion.*

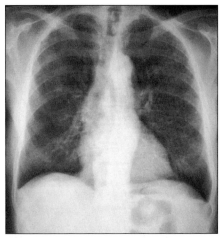

Fig. 6.56 *Chest X-ray in miliary tuberculosis.*

infection or may result from reactivation. Patients with tuberculous effusions usually have a cough and fever. Some may lose weight and have chest pain. Rarely the effusions are so large as to cause breathlessness. Although effusions will resolve spontaneously over the next few months, there is a high risk of later disease.

If a patient with a past history of TB or with evidence of TB elsewhere in the body presents with a pleural effusion, it is likely that they have a tuberculosis effusion. Diagnosis rests on demonstrating the presence of *M. tuberculosis*. Acid-fast bacilli are rarely seen on direct microscopy but may be cultured in up to half of cases. Pleural biopsy increases the yield, particularly if more than one biopsy is taken.

MILIARY TUBERCULOSIS

When *M. tuberculosis* disseminates haematogenously, patients may become extremely unwell. Miliary disease is more common in children and in immunocompromised patients. The organisms particularly seed to the bone marrow, liver, lungs and eyes. The lesions produced on the chest X-ray look like small millet seeds; hence the term 'miliary' (Fig. 6.56). Although many patients are acutely sick, others have an indolent disease and may present with a fever of unknown origin.

Diagnosis can be difficult. Nonspecific features such as abnormal liver function tests and mild pancytopenia are occasionally found. Although the chest X-ray may show classical miliary shadowing, it can be normal, particularly in the first few months of disease. The organism may be demonstrated by examination and culture of bone marrow or liver. With new lysis–centrifugation blood culture techniques, blood culture of *M. tuberculosis* is possible.

TUBERCULIN SKIN TESTING

Using tuberculin protein as an antigen, skin testing of delayed-type hypersensitivity may give some information about exposure to *M. tuberculosis*. The Heaf test or the Mantoux test may be used, and a positive test is interpreted as meaning that the patient has cell-mediated immunity to tuberculin protein. This may be the result of past infection, active disease or previous bacillus Calmette–Guérin (BCG) vaccination. In the Mantoux test, which is the easiest to perform, 1 tuberculin unit (0.1 ml of a 1:10,000 solution of tuberculin) is injected

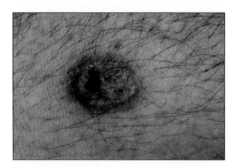

Fig. 6.57 *Positive Mantoux test.*

intradermally into the flexor part of the forearm. The test is 'read' at 48–72 hours and is deemed positive if there is palpable induration with a diameter of more than 5 mm (**Fig. 6.57**). If it is negative, the test can be repeated using a 1:1000 solution (10 tuberculin units).

Interpretation of tuberculin skin tests can be difficult, particularly in the setting of previous BCG vaccination or in highly endemic areas. It is unreliable as a diagnostic test for active infection because up to 25% of cases of active pulmonary tuberculosis may be negative.

TREATMENT OF TUBERCULOSIS

The tubercle bacillus is slow growing and some organisms may be naturally resistant to certain antituberculous drugs. Successful treatment requires multiple drug combinations. This increases bacterial killing and minimizes the chances of resistant mutants surviving. At least three drugs should be given initially, although only two may be required for consolidation treatment. The most common regimen involves rifampicin, isoniazid and pyrazinamide. The first two are given for the duration of therapy (usually 6 months) with pyrazinamide given only for the first 2 months. If resistance is suspected (e.g. in immigrants from endemic areas or those previously treated for tuberculosis), a fourth drug should be added, usually ethambutol.

Treatment is required for at least 6 months to ensure cure, so attention to ensuring compliance is essential. This is best done by directly observed therapy, which has been shown to be highly cost effective in a variety of settings. Whenever possible, specimens should be obtained for culture and antibiotic sensitivity before starting therapy so that drug resistance can be recognized early.

Good tuberculosis control programmes need, in addition to well-supervised treatment, effective contact tracing and rigorous chasing of defaulters from treatment. About 10% of close contacts of patients with open (sputum-positive) tuberculosis become infected. The spectre of multiple-drug resistant *M. tuberculosis* is an increasing problem in some countries.

The role of adjunctive corticosteroid therapy is usually controversial. Although it has been demonstrated to be of use in pericardial disease, there is no good evidence to support its role in pulmonary disease. Corticosteroids are sometimes used, however, in large pleural effusions and in very ill patients.

chapter 7

Central Nervous System Infections

INTRODUCTION

Central nervous system infections, including bacterial and viral meningitis and viral encephalitis, are major causes of morbidity and mortality. In the USA about 15,000 cases are reported annually, with a case fatality rate of 10–15%. It has been estimated that in underdeveloped countries such as The Gambia, 2% of all children born will die of meningitis before they reach 5 years of age.

BACTERIAL MENINGITIS

Bacterial meningitis usually arises from a bacteraemic event following colonization or infection at another focus. Colonization of the nasopharynx with silent bacteraemia or overt infection elsewhere, such as otitis media, pneumonia or sinusitis, may be apparent.

CLINICAL FEATURES

The principle signs and symptoms of bacterial meningitis – headache, fever and stiff neck – are seen in about 90% of patients. These findings may be absent in young children or the elderly. Brudzinski's sign – forceful anteflexion of the neck resulting in involuntary flexion of the knees or hips – and Kerning's sign – resistance to extension when extending the knee – may be absent in about half of all patients. Altered mental status, vomiting and seizures may occur. There may be focal neurological findings and evidence of infection at distant sites. In infants bulging fontanelles may be present.

DIAGNOSIS

The cerebrospinal fluid (CSF) typically has an increased intracranial pressure associated with increased protein and leucocyte concentrations with hypoglycorrhachia (decreased

Typical cerebrospinal fluid profile in types of meningitis

Entity	Cells per mm³	Differential	Protein (g/l)	Glucose (mmol/l)
Bacterial meningitis	200–20,000	Polymorphonucleocytes	1.0–10*	<2.5
Aseptic meningitis	100–1000	Lymphocytes	0.5–1.0	3.3
Mycobacterial infection	100–500	Lymphocytes	1.0–2.0*	<2.8
Fungal infection	10–200	Lymphocytes	0.5–2.0*	<2.2

* in cases of cerebrospinal fluid blockage, protein may be markedly increased

Fig. 7.1 *Typical CSF profile in types of meningitis.*

glucose in the CSF) (**Fig. 7.1**). Diagnosis of the causative organism generally rests on Gram stain and culture of CSF, which detects about 70–80% of organisms. Other studies, such as latex agglutination for antigens in the CSF may be useful, especially in patients who have received previous antimicrobial therapy.

The most common pathogens are *Streptococcus pneumoniae* and *Neisseria meningitidis*. The use of *Haemophilus influenzae* vaccine has dramatically decreased the frequency of *H. influenzae* meningitis in developed countries, although this organism is still the most common cause of meningitis worldwide. *H. influenzae*, a Gram-negative coccobacillus, may be particularly difficult to detect on Gram stain (**Fig. 7.2**). The Gram stain characteristics of *S. pneumoniae* (**Fig. 7.3**) and *N. meningitidis* (**Fig. 7.4**) are sufficiently distinctive to differentiate these organisms.

In about 50% of cases of meningococcal meningitis, widespread petaechiae may be present (**Fig. 7.5**).

Among elderly, pregnant and immunocompromised patients there are additional organisms that deserve consideration – *Listeria monocytogenes*, Gram-negative bacilli and *Cryptococcus neoformans* (see Chapter 13). *L. monocytogenes* is a Gram-positive rod that causes infection in immunocompromised and pregnant patients – meningitis is one clinical manifestation. In *Listeria* meningitis, the Gram stain of the CSF is often negative, although Gram-positive rods may be seen (**Fig. 7.6**). Among immunocompromised patients *C. neoformans* becomes an important cause of meningitis. Diagnosis can be made by India ink exam of CSF or latex agglutination testing for antigen in the CSF.

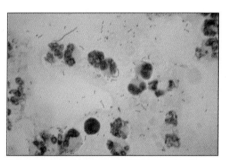

Fig. 7.2 Haemophilus influenzae *in Gram stain of cerebrospinal fluid.*

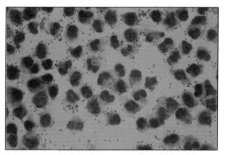

Fig. 7.3 Streptococcus pneumoniae *in Gram stain of cerebrospinal fluid.*

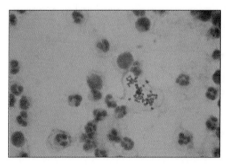

Fig. 7.4 Neisseria meningitidis *in Gram stain of cerebrospinal fluid.*

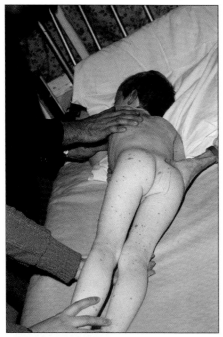

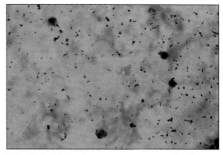

Fig. 7.6 Listeria monocytogenes *in Gram stain of cerebrospinal fluid.*

Fig. 7.5 *Petaechiae in child with meningococcal meningitis and meningococcaemia.*

Neonatal meningitis is a distinct clinical entity, most frequently caused by *Escherichia coli* or group B streptococci. The diagnosis may be especially difficult because signs in neonates may be very nonspecific.

MANAGEMENT

The management of bacterial meningitis requires rapid assessment and therapy. Focal neurological findings may require the use of neuroimaging with a CT scan or MRI of the brain to rule out a space occupying lesion. The time from evaluation to antimicrobial therapy should not exceed 30 minutes. Lumbar puncture for CSF assessment should be performed and empiric antibiotics, aimed at the most common pathogens, should be given (**Fig. 7.7**). Because of poor penetration through the blood–brain barrier, the antibiotics should be given intravenously in high doses.

The use of corticosteroids as adjunctive therapy has been advocated in children because it has been shown that they reduce long-term neurological sequelae of meningitis due to *H. influenzae* type B. Such additional therapy is considered more controversial in adults, especially in those with pneumococcal meningitis.

INFECTIONS OF CENTRAL NERVOUS SYSTEM SHUNTS

There is a common type of meningitis that complicates the placement of CSF shunts placement – CSF shunt meningitis. These infections occur as a result of contamination of the shunt by local bacterial contamination or bacteraemic seeding. Frequent symptoms are

Recommendations for empiric therapy of bacterial meningitis

Age	Standard therapy	Alternative therapy
0–3 weeks	Ampicillin + cefotaxime	Ampicillin + aminoglycoside
4–12 weeks	Cefotaxime or ceftriaxone + ampicillin ± vancomycin	
3 months–18 years	Third-generation cephalosporin ± vancomycin	Ampicillin, chloramphenicol or a combination of both
18–60 years	Third-generation cephalosporin ± ampicillin ± vancomycin	Penicillin G, chloramphenicol
>60 years	Third-generation cephalosporin ± ampicillin ± vancomycin	Ampicillin + aminoglycoside, co-trimoxazole

Fig. 7.7 Recommendations for empiric therapy of bacterial meningitis.

fever and headache, with nausea, vomiting and change in mental status. There may be no pain at the shunt site. The organisms causing this infection are typically of low virulence, such as *Staphylococcus epidermidis* and *Propionibacterium acnes* (**Fig. 7.8**).

BRAIN ABSCESS

Brain abscesses typically occur as a result of infection elsewhere, such as sinusitis or bacteraemia, or as a complication of neurological surgery. Depending on the size and location of the mass lesion, neurological findings may be diverse or nonexistent. The microbiology of brain abscess is typically mixed, with combinations of aerobic and anaerobic organisms (**Fig. 7.9**). Microaerophilic streptococci, such as *Streptococcus milleri*, are very commonly found. Occasionally, *Staphylococcus aureus* may be the pathogen, typically as a complication of *S. aureus* endocarditis. Post-neurosurgical infections may lead to an epidural abscess or empyema in addition to a brain abscess. The organisms may be more indolent, such as coagulase-negative staphylococci and corynebacteria. In immunocompromised patients, brain abscesses may be caused by *Nocardia* spp. (**Fig. 7.10**) or by fungal pathogens such as *Aspergillus* spp. or disseminated candidiasis.

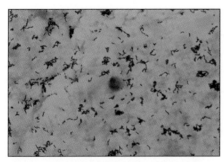

Fig. 7.8 *Gram stain of* Propionibacterium acnes *causing infection of a cerebrospinal fluid shunt.*

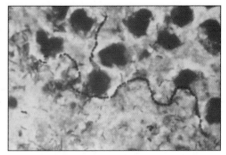

Fig. 7.9 *Gram stain of brain abscess caused by mixed aerobic and anaerobic pathogens.*

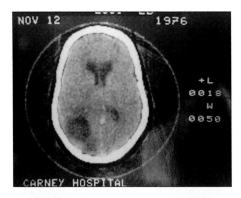

Fig. 7.10 *CT scan of a patient with a* Nocardia *brain abscess.*

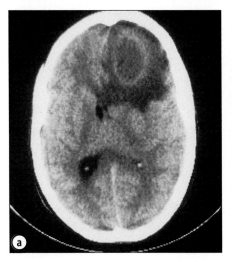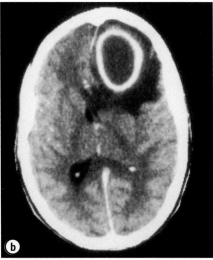

Fig. 7.11 *CT scan of the brain with contrast showing brain abscess (a) pre-contrast;* *(b) post-contrast.*

Diagnosis rests on CT scanning showing a ring enhancing lesion (**Fig. 7.11**) followed by aspiration of purulent material. Parenteral antibiotics for 4–6 weeks are required to effect a cure. Aspiration of purulent material either at surgery or under stereotactic guidance by CT scan may be required.

INFECTION OF THE SUBDURAL AND EPIDURAL SPACE

There are several other infections of the central nervous system whose manifestations occur as a result of anatomic displacement of structures, namely subdural infections and epidural infections.

Infection of the subdural space typically occurs as a result of extension of osteomyelitis of the skull with an accompanying epidural abscess (**Fig. 7.12**). A variety of organisms, such as staphylococci, streptococci or mixed aerobic and anaerobic organisms, cause these infections. Alteration in mental status and focal neurological deficits are common. Rapid progression may ensue. Assessment using CT scan or MRI (**Fig. 7.13**) may be necessary to localize the lesion for surgical intervention, which is often necessary.

An epidural abscess may occur from direct extension of a subdural empyema. Most cases are associated with frontal sinusitis, craniotomy or mastoiditis. Headache and focal neurological findings may be present. Diagnosis can be made by MRI with gadolinium enhancement and aspiration of infected material. The aetiological organisms are the same as those seen in subdural empyema.

Spinal epidural abscesses frequently occur as a result of metastatic infection from elsewhere in the body. Infection may reach the epidural space via the bloodstream or by contiguous spread from adjacent vertebral osteomyelitis (**Fig. 7.14**) – or the space may be seeded following traumatic injury (such as spinal anaesthesia, lumbar puncture or back surgery). *S. aureus* is the most common aetiological agent, but many other pathogens may be causative. Plain X-ray of the spine, CT scan, MRI (**Fig. 7.15**) or myelography may define the lesion. Because of the danger of spinal cord necrosis, surgical drainage is necessary.

ASEPTIC MENINGITIS

Aseptic meningitis refers to the syndrome of meningitis in which there are no bacteria and the lymphocyte is the predominant cell in the CSF. This syndrome is typically due to

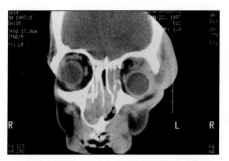

Fig. 7.12 *MRI scan showing osteomyelitis of the skull and accompanying subdural empyema.*

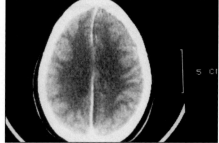

Fig. 7.13 *CT scan showing a subdural empyema displacing falx anteriorly.*

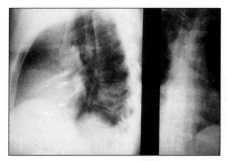

Fig. 7.14 *Plain X-ray of thoracic spine showing osteomyelitis with accompanying spinal epidural abscess.*

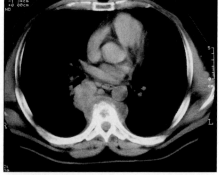

Fig. 7.15 *CT scan of the spine showing a spinal epidural abscess.*

infection with enteroviruses. Other pathogens such as *Mycobacterium tuberculosis*, *Borrelia burgdorferi* (the causative agent of Lyme disease), *Treponema pallidum* (the causative agent of syphilis) and other viruses such as HIV may also cause lymphocytic CSF and present as aseptic meningitis.

In meningitis caused by enteroviruses, the CSF characteristically shows a lymphocytic pleocytosis, with modest elevations in protein, and normal to only slightly low levels of glucose. Diagnosis rests on absence of evidence of bacterial or other pathogens such as cryptococci, *M. tuberculosis*, *T. pallidum* and *B. burgdorferi*. Enteroviruses can be cultured from cerebrospinal fluid, stool or throat wash specimens. Although serology for enteroviruses is available, its use should be discouraged owing to the ubiquitous nature of these viruses. Many people have pre-existing antibody to one or more enteroviruses; furthermore, there are a large number of serotypes to be tested for. Recent studies with the polymerase chain reaction have shown that it is useful in making a diagnosis of central nervous system infection due to enteroviruses.

Therapy for viral-associated aseptic meningitis is purely supportive unless infection can be demonstrated to be due to HIV, cytomegalovirus or herpes simplex virus (HSV), for which specific therapy may be useful.

CHRONIC MENINGITIS

There are a number of infectious agents that may cause chronic meningitis. Granulomatous processes (e.g. tuberculosis) and chronic fungal disease (e.g. histoplasmosis, coccidioidomycosis or blastomycosis) may cause chronic meningitis. *B. burgdorferi* infection may also cause chronic central nervous system involvement, as may syphilis and brucellosis.

Cysticercosis may present as a seizure disorder with or without a meningitic component. CT scans of the head (**Fig. 7.16**) or even plain X-rays of the skull may show scattered calcifications, which, when present in someone from an endemic area, are virtually diagnostic.

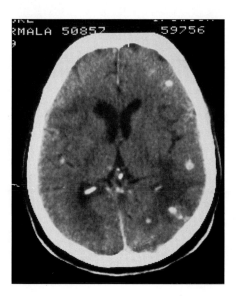

Fig. 7.16 *CT scan showing calcification in a patient with cerebral cysticercosis.*

VIRAL ENCEPHALITIS

Viral encephalitis is characterized by altered mental status and altered personality, generally with the presence of seizures. As with aseptic meningitis, the CSF is characterized by mononuclear cell predominance; however, in viral encephalitis the degree of cellularity, the level of protein and the opening pressure are generally elevated to a much greater extent.

The most common cause of fatal, nonepidemic viral encephalitis is herpes simplex virus (HSV). HSV encephalitis is characterized by focal haemorrhagic necrosis of the temporal lobe (**Fig. 7.17**). The clinical presentation is frequently acute, with altered mentation, focal neurological findings and seizures. Diagnosis may require brain biopsy, in which the pathologic evidence of the virus may be present (**Fig. 7.18**). Direct immunofluorescence or viral culture may confirm the diagnosis. Newer techniques, such as use of the polymerase chain reaction on CSF to detect HSV genomes, have also been employed to make the diagnosis.

Early therapy with aciclovir can be curative; at the very least it decreases morbidity and mortality. A number of other infections and noninfectious processes can mimic HSV encephalitis, and therefore it is important to rule out this specific agent.

Epidemic forms of viral encephalitis are typically due to arthropod-borne viruses (arboviruses) (**Fig. 7.19**). These infections occur in the summer, are transmitted by mosquitoes and have very specific geographical distributions. Findings are generally nonspecific with loss of consciousness, seizures and fever. Diagnosis may be made by antibody studies of serum or CSF or by isolating the virus. Unfortunately, there is no effective therapy for any of the arboviral agents.

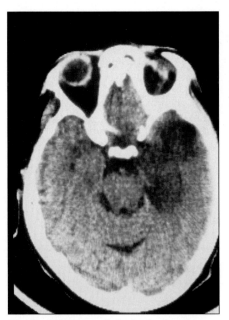

Fig. 7.17 *CT scan of the brain showing herpes simplex virus involvement of the temporal lobe.*

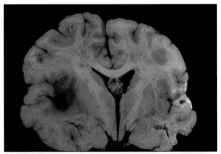

Fig. 7.18 *Herpes simplex encephalitis: section of brain showing haemorrhage in right temporal lobe.*

Arboviral infections causing encephalitis according to vector and geographical distribution		
Class of agent	**Distribution**	**Vector**
Alphaviruses		
Eastern equine (encephalitis virus)	Americas	Mosquito
Venezuelan equine (encephalitis virus)	Americas	Mosquito
Western equine (encephalitis virus)	Americas	Mosquito
Flaviviruses		
Japanese (B encephalitis virus)	Asia, Pacific	Mosquito
Kyasanur Forest (virus)	India	Tick
Louping ill (virus)	UK	Tick
Murray Valley (encephalitis virus)	Australia, New Guinea	Mosquito
Powassan virus	North America, Russia	Tick
St Louis (encephalitis virus)	Americas	Mosquito
Tick-borne (encephalitis virus)	Europe, Asia	Tick
Bunyaviruses		
Rift Valley fever (virus)	Africa	Mosquito
California	USA	Mosquito

Fig. 7.19 *Arboviral infections causing encephalitis according to vector and geographical distribution.*

RABIES

Rabies, a rare form of viral encephalitis in the developed world, is a very common problem in developing countries. Animal bites from a rabid animal may transmit the infection, which has a long incubation period of weeks or even months. Progressive neurological deterioration with hydrophobia may ensue. The CSF is only minimally reactive, with a modest elevation in cells and elevated protein. Once disease develops it is almost invariably fatal; very rare cases of survival have been reported, but all of these have had significant neurological deficits.

Diagnosis can be made by detection of immunofluorescence of tissues for rabies virus antigens on skin biopsy, corneal smears or brain biopsy. The pathogenic changes in the brain are quite distinct, with the presence of cytoplasmic Negri bodies being the pathognomonic neuronal change (**Fig. 7.20**).

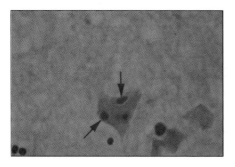

Fig. 7.20 *Pathology of a brain infected with rabies virus, showing Negri bodies.*

There is no therapy. Prevention of contact with rabid animals and pre-exposure immunization are necessary to prevent transmission. Post-exposure vaccination is useful following a bite.

OTHER BACTERIAL INFECTIONS OF THE CENTRAL NERVOUS SYSTEM

TUBERCULOSIS

Tuberculosis occasionally presents as a central nervous system infection. In children this infection typically presents as one manifestation of a systemic progressive disease. In adults with *M. tuberculosis* infection of the central nervous system, neurological abnormalities may be the only presenting features. Ocular palsies predominate.

Typical CSF findings include 300–500 lymphocytes per mm³, elevated protein and modestly decreased glucose. Cerebrospinal fluid acid-fast smears are rarely positive; CSF cultures for *M. tuberculosis* are positive in about 50% of cases. Attempts at molecular techniques and antigen detection within the CSF show promise but are not generally clinically available.

Therapy with antituberculosis drugs should be employed in accordance with general treatment of *M. tuberculosis* infection. In addition, corticosteroids have been shown to be useful as adjunctive therapy to decrease the amount of inflammation and reduce chronic neurological sequelae.

LYME DISEASE

In some regions of the world infection with *B. burgdorferi* (Lyme disease) is a common form of aseptic meningitis. Central nervous system involvement typically presents with a triad of paraesthesiae, cranial nerve palsies (especially of the seventh cranial nerve) and peripheral neuropathy. Progression to a form of chronic meningitis or meningoencephalitis may occur.

The CSF is characterized by a lymphocytic pleocytosis, mildly abnormal protein and normal or slightly decreased glucose. Therapy requires intravenous ceftriaxone for a prolonged period of time.

CREUTZFELDT–JAKOB DISEASE

This rare form of encephalopathy is caused by agents called prions. These transmissible agents form prion proteins, which are resistant to heat, chemicals and irradiation. Microscopy of the brain in Creutzfeldt–Jakob disease (CJD) reveals a spongiform appearance with little or no inflammatory response (**Fig. 7.21**) – hence the name

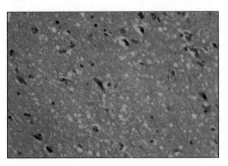

Fig. 7.21 *Pathology of the brain of a patient with Creutzfeldt–Jakob disease.*

'spongiform encephalopathy'. Transmission of this rare agent in humans has occurred from corneal grafts, improper sterilization of stereotactic needles and pooled human growth hormone. CJD is very similar to the disease kuru, a fatal neurological disease with cerebellar signs that is seen in Papua New Guinea. A recently described variant, bovine spongiform encephalopathy (BSE) has been described in the UK. Compared to classic CJD, this new variant of CJD (nvCJD) occurs at a younger age (usually less than 30 years) and follows a more rapidly progressive course. The human illness has been linked to 'mad cow disease' in the UK and may be due to consumption of contaminated beef.

OTHER CHRONIC VIRAL INFECTIONS OF THE CENTRAL NERVOUS SYSTEM

Another form of a chronic viral infection of the central nervous system is that due to chronic progressive disease from measles infection and measles vaccination or, very rarely, as a complication of subacute sclerosing panencephalitis.

Chronic progressive rubella or JC virus infection (a polyoma virus) may also give rise to chronic neurological disease.

In patients infected with HIV, progressive multifocal leucoencephalopathy has a distinctive appearance on CT scan (**Fig. 7.22**).

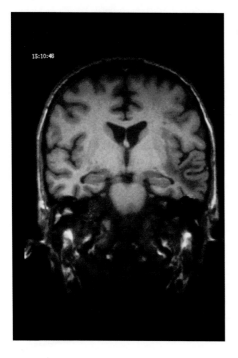

Fig. 7.22 *Progressive multifocal leucoencephalopathy: MRI (T_1-weighted image) showing white matter changes in the left temporal lobe.*

BOTULISM

Botulism is a disease characterized by descending weakness and paralysis accompanied by dysphagia, diplopia, vomiting, vertigo and respiratory failure. The disease is caused by ingestion of preformed toxin elaborated by the organism *Clostridium botulinum*. This toxin is produced when canned or preserved foods are contaminated by spores, which subsequently generate toxin. The ingestion of toxin leads to blockage of acetylcholine release in nerve synapses. Diagnosis is based on clinical suspicion and demonstration of toxin in food, serum or stool. Treatment is supportive, along with administration of antitoxin. A rare variant, seen in infants who ingest honey contaminated with *C. botulinum*, may lead to generalized weakness and the 'floppy baby' syndrome.

POSTINFECTIOUS SYNDROMES

ACUTE INFLAMMATORY POLYNEUROPATHY

Acute inflammation and demyelination may occur as a postinfectious complication. The Guillain–Barré syndrome often follows:

- a respiratory illness, such as infection with *Mycoplasma pneumoniae*;
- a viral illness, such as cytomegalovirus or Epstein–Barr virus; or
- gastrointestinal ailments, such as infection with *Campylobacter* spp. or *Salmonella* spp.

Symptoms are characterized by paraesthesias in the lower extremities followed by weakness in the feet and lower legs. Ascending paralysis may lead to respiratory failure. The CSF is characterized by a lymphocytic pleocytosis with elevated protein levels. Management is supportive, with plasmapheresis, immunosuppression or intravenous immunoglobulin used as adjunctive therapy.

TRANSVERSE MYELITIS

Transverse myelitis, like Guillain-Barré syndrome, may follow a relatively minor infection. Myelitis may simulate transection of the cord, with limb weakness, loss of bowel and bladder control, and sensory dysfunction at the level of the lesion. A number of infections can cause a transverse myelitis, including Epstein–Barr virus, measles, rubella, varicella-zoster virus, *B. burgdorferi*, human T-lymphotropic virus type I, HIV and a number of other pathogens.

NEURITIS

Neuritis is an inflammatory process involving peripheral nerves. Leprosy, trypanosomes and microsporidia can cause a direct inflammatory response. Bacterial toxins such as tetanus, diphtheria or botulinum can also cause neuritis. Many of the pathogens that cause transverse myelitis may cause direct nerve injury as well.

chapter 8

Ocular Infections

INFECTIONS OF THE EYELIDS

BLEPHARITIS

Blepharitis is an inflammation of the eyelids. It may be acute or chronic, is usually bilateral and may be seen in association with conjunctivitis. Some cases are allergic in origin or are related to seborrhoeic dermatitis, but some are secondary to staphylococcal infection. Many cases are due to coagulase-negative staphylococci; others are due to *Staphylococcus aureus*. The majority are low-grade chronic infections. Patients usually have mild irritation with some diffuse redness of the edges of the eyelids. There may be a fibrinous exudate that forms crusts at the bases of the lashes (**Fig. 8.1**).

Treatment relies on improving local hygiene to keep the eyelids clean. Topical antibiotic treatment may be required for several weeks, usually with mupirocin ointment. In some cases that are associated with rosacea, systemic tetracycline may be used.

HORDEOLUM

Hordeolae, or sties, may occur in the anterior, or external, part of the lid as a result of staphylococcal infection of the glands of Zeis (**Fig. 8.2**). Internal, or posterior, sties involve the meibomian glands. Infections are usually acute, with pain and redness in the lid followed by the formation of small abscesses that are visible at the lid margin. Meibomian gland infections are less likely to 'point' and may present more like a limited cellulitis of the lid. Sometimes chronic inflammation leads to the formation of a chalazion (a granuloma within the meibomian gland).

External sties often burst and resolve spontaneously but they may require local antibiotic ointment. Internal sties may resolve with topical treatment but they sometimes require systemic antistaphylococcal therapy. Chalazions that do not resolve spontaneously may regress with local steroid treatment.

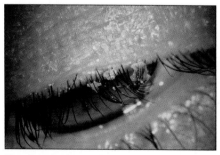

Fig. 8.1 *Scaly exudate on the eyelashes in blepharitis.*

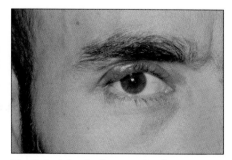

Fig. 8.2 *A hordeolum, or sty, due to* Staphylococcus aureus *infection.*

CONJUNCTIVITIS

Infections of the conjunctiva are usually bilateral and present with a gritty sensation in the eye and no impairment of vision. The eyes often look infected and there may be associated exudate and matting of the lids (**Fig. 8.3**). This condition needs to be distinguished from keratitis and iritis.

BACTERIAL CONJUNCTIVITIS

Most cases are due to Gram-positive cocci, predominantly *S. aureus*. Epidemics caused by *Streptococcus pneumoniae* may occur. Gram-negative infections can occur, especially in abnormal eyes or in patients who are unconscious. *Haemophilus influenzae* type b used to cause a large number of infections in children but the incidence has declined after the introduction of vaccination. Occasional epidemics due to *Haemophilus aegypticus* occur. Gonococcal infection of the conjunctiva may occur in neonates following exposure in the birth canal (ophthalmia neonatorum), and adults may get gonococcal conjunctivitis through sexual contact.

Treatment of bacterial conjunctivitis hastens recovery. Swabs and corneal scrapings may help diagnosis but most cases are treated empirically. Eye drops or ointments containing either chloramphenicol, aminoglycosides, vancomycin or fluoroquinolones are all usually effective. The only exception to topical therapy is gonococcal ophthalmia neonatorum when systemic therapy may be required.

CHLAMYDIAL CONJUNCTIVITIS

Chlamydia trachomatis serotypes A, B and C cause trachoma, an important cause of blindness in the tropics. Serotypes D–K cause an inclusion conjunctivitis. In trachoma, initial symptoms may be minimal during the period follicles appear on the conjunctivae. With time, a keratitis ensues and further damage results in abnormal eyelids, secondary trauma and bacterial infection. Inclusion conjunctivitis is usually sexually acquired in association with nongonococcal urethritis. There is usually a low-grade, chronic inflammation of the conjunctivae with formation of large follicles (**Fig. 8.4**). Neonates may get a similar infection which, if untreated, may lead on to keratitis.

Trachoma is usually treated with systemic tetracycline in adults, but children and pregnant women should receive topical therapy. Antibiotics are usually required for 3–4 weeks. Inclusion conjunctivitis and chlamydial ophthalmia neonatorum are treated by systemic tetracycline; pregnant women and children should receive erythromycin.

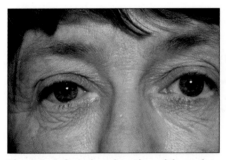

Fig. 8.3 *Infected conjunctiva with exudate in bacterial conjunctivitis.*

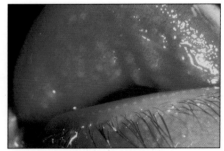

Fig. 8.4 *Eyelid in early trachoma.*

VIRAL CONJUNCTIVITIS

In developed countries, most cases of conjunctivitis are viral and most are due to adenovirus infection. Infections can be unilateral or bilateral and, unlike bacterial conjunctivitis, there is often enlargement of preauricular lymph nodes (**Fig. 8.5**).

Pharyngoconjunctival fever is due to adenovirus types 3, 4 or 7 and is seen mainly in children. There is mild systemic upset with fever and sore throat along with a watery discharge from the affected eyes.

Epidemic keratoconjunctivitis is due to types 8 or 19 and is highly contagious. Adults are affected and outbreaks are common. It is more severe than the childhood infections and the cornea may be involved in severe cases.

Acute haemorrhagic conjunctivitis describes a severe bilateral infection that may occur in outbreaks. Coxsackievirus is the most common cause.

Other viruses may cause conjunctivitis, the most important of which is herpes simplex virus (HSV). Infections with HSV are more common in children and may cause a keratitis.

Most cases of viral conjunctivitis are treated symptomatically and resolve over a few weeks. HSV conjunctivitis should be treated with topical aciclovir.

CORNEAL INFECTIONS

These are more serious than conjunctival infections because they may lead to ulceration and scarring of the cornea.

BACTERIAL KERATITIS

Most of these infections require some defect in the corneal epithelium because the healthy cornea is relatively resistant to infection. Minor trauma from entropion, contact lenses, foreign bodies or dryness from thyroid eye disease may all predispose to bacterial infection. The most common organisms are staphylococci, streptococci (including the pneumococcus), Enterobacteriaceae and *Pseudomonas aeruginosa*.

Bacterial keratitis may be fulminant, in which case patients present with pain and redness, photophobia and discharge from the eye. In addition to obvious erythema of the eye and eyelid oedema, the cornea may have a white, shaggy infiltrate and appear hazy. There may be a hypopyon – a layer of white cells collecting in the lower part of the anterior chamber (**Fig. 8.6**).

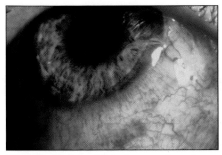

Fig. 8.5 *Conjunctivitis due to adenovirus infection.*

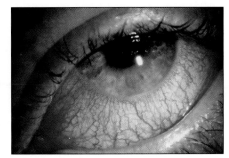

Fig. 8.6 *A small hypopyon.*

Examination with a slit lamp may reveal a corneal ulcer. A scraping should be taken from the cornea for Gram stain and culture, but treatment should be started empirically with broad-spectrum topical antibiotics given in high dose at short intervals; treatment can be modified later on the basis of culture results. The pupil should be dilated to prevent synechia formation.

VIRAL KERATITIS

Herpes simplex virus is the most common cause of viral keratitis and HSV keratitis is the most severe of the viral keratides. Children rarely develop keratitis as a consequence of HSV conjunctivitis; most cases are in adults and probably represent reactivation of latent infection. The keratitis is usually monocular and causes dendritic ulcers (**Fig. 8.7**). This infection may lead to a uveitis. HSV keratitis should be treated with topical aciclovir and some cases require epithelial debridement.

Varicella-zoster virus infection of the cornea may occur in the setting of shingles affecting the ophthalmic or maxillary divisions of the fifth cranial nerve. Although dendritic ulcers are less common than with HSV keratitis, corneal scarring can occur (**Fig. 8.8**). Patients require systemic antiviral therapy as well as topical treatment.

A host of other viruses rarely cause keratitis. Adenovirus infections may be spread in ophthalmology clinics via contaminated equipment such as tonometers.

FUNGAL KERATITIS

Fungi are rare causes of keratitis, *Aspergillus* spp. being the most common. Other fungi include *Fusarium* spp. and *Candida* spp. Primary fungal infections are unusual in the absence of trauma or some form of immunosuppression. Clinically, there is usually an infiltrate in the corneal stroma with feathery borders. There may be multiple satellite lesions and a small hypopyon. Diagnosis is difficult. If fungi are suspected, corneal scrapings and, sometimes, a corneal biopsy is required to obtain specimens for culture and histology. Treatment is also difficult; natamycin is used topically in North America but dilute (0.15% solution) amphotericin B may be equally effective. Topical flucytosine may be effective for yeast infections, and the role of the newer imidazoles is not yet established.

AMOEBIC KERATITIS

Rarely, in people who wear soft contact lenses, a keratitis due to *Acanthamoeba* spp. (usually *Acanthamoeba polyphaga or Acanthamoeba castellani*) may occur.

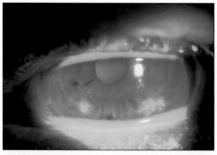

Fig. 8.7 *Dendritic ulcer (fluroscein staining) due to herpes simplex virus (HSV) infection.*

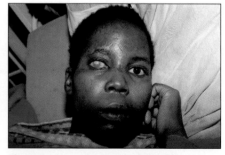

Fig. 8.8 *Corneal scarring following ophthalmic zoster with keratitis.*

INFECTIOUS ENDOPHTHALMITIS

Most cases of endophthalmitis now follow eye surgery, although some result from trauma and a few from metastatic spread from a distant focus.

POSTOPERATIVE ENDOPHTHALMITIS
Early disease occurs within 2 weeks of surgery, with up to 60% of cases being caused by staphylococci, both coagulase-negative and coagulase-positive staphylococci. There is usually acute pain and poor visual acuity. Examination reveals anterior chamber inflammation, including hypopyon. Inflammation of the vitreous humour is common.

Late disease (more than 2 weeks after surgery) is most likely to be due to coagulase-negative staphylococci, fungi or *Propionobacterium* spp. Infection with *Propionobacterium* spp. is a common sequel to lens implantation and presents with white foci of infection within the lens capsule. Staphylococcal infection is often associated with hypopyon and vitritis (**Fig. 8.9**). Fungal infections are characterized by progressive white infiltrates in the anterior chamber, sometimes referred to as a 'string of pearls' appearance. These infections may present relatively slowly with declining visual acuity.

Some patients develop conjunctival 'blebs' after surgery for cataract or glaucoma. Such blebs may act as a route for infection to spread into the aqueous humour. Streptococci and *Haemophilus* spp. are most commonly implicated in such infections.

ENDOPHTHALMITIS FOLLOWING TRAUMA
Endophthalmitis may follow trauma with an object that is contaminated with plant or soil debris. A common organism involved is *Bacillus cereus*, although streptococci and staphylococci may also be implicated.

ENDOGENOUS ENDOPHTHALMITIS
Some patients who are bacteraemic or fungaemic may have septic emboli to the eye, resulting in endophthalmitis. *S. aureus* and streptococci are the most common bacteria. About 10% of patients with candidaemia may develop fungal endophthalmitis at some stage (**Fig. 8.10**).

DIAGNOSIS
Accurate microbiological diagnosis is essential for optimal management of endophthalmitis. Samples should be obtained from both the anterior and posterior chambers and cultured appropriately. Patients with endogenous endophthalmitis should be assessed for distant foci of infection, such as endocarditis.

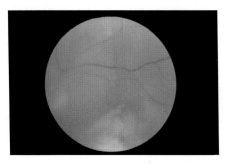

Fig. 8.9 *Endophthalmitis due to* **Staphylococcus aureus** *infection.*

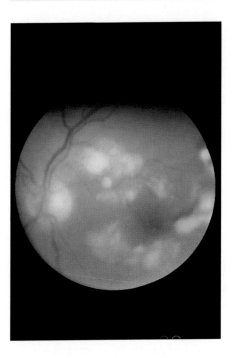

Fig. 8.10 *Snowball appearance in candidal endophthalmitis.*

TREATMENT

In postoperative endophthalmitis, empiric treatment should begin as soon as samples have been taken. Reasonable treatments are either vancomycin plus amikacin or vancomycin plus ceftazidime, both given as intravitreal injections. Intraocular dexamethasone is also recommended by some authorities. Vitrectomy is reserved for severe cases and for fungal infection.

Infections with *Propionobacterium acnes* in the setting of lens implants require complete excision of the lens capsule along with intravitreal vancomycin and dexamethasone.

Vancomycin plus ceftazidime is recommended for endophthalmitis secondary to trauma or conjunctival blebs. If conjunctival blebs are present, therapeutic vitrectomy may be required.

Endogenous endophthalmitis caused by infection elsewhere should be treated with systemic antimicrobials as well as with intravitreal therapy. The distant focus should be removed, if possible.

CHOROIDORETINITIS

Most cases of choroidoretinitis are due to viral infections although some are caused by parasites.

VIRAL RETINITIS

The majority of cases are caused by herpesviruses. The primary symptom is decreased visual acuity, sometimes preceded by 'floaters'. HSV type 1 is usually more severe in primary infections than in reactivations and is often associated with encephalitis. There are usually retinal haemorrhages and oedema, and retinal detachment may occur. In cases of encephalitis, retinal changes may easily be overlooked as the patients are usually severely ill. HSV type 2 infection predominantly occurs in neonates born to mothers with active genital herpes or cervical shedding. Retinitis may occur in up to 20% of infected neonates. Increasingly, HSV type 2 is a cause of encephalitis in adults and there may be an associated retinitis.

Cytomegalovirus (CMV) is a particular problem in immunocompromised patients, especially those with the acquired immunodeficiency syndrome (AIDS). The retina has a characteristic appearance with vasculitis, haemorrhage and exudates, leading to retinal necrosis (**Fig. 8.11**). Epstein-Barr virus is a rare cause of retinitis.

Varicella-zoster virus (VZV) may affect the eye in a variety of ways. Retinitis is very rare in chickenpox except in the setting of congenital infection. However, posterior uveitis and retinitis may complicate ophthalmic zoster.

Rarely, other viruses are associated with retinitis (**Fig. 8.12**).

TREATMENT

Retinitis due to HSV or VZV requires systemic treatment with high dose parenteral aciclovir. CMV retinitis in the setting of HIV is frequently treated with systemic ganciclovir, or foscarnet or, more recently, cidofovir. Intravitreal therapy is also effective.

ACUTE RETINAL NECROSIS SYNDROME

Acute retinal necrosis syndrome is a distinct clinical entity that is most commonly associated with VZV infections but it also occurs with HSV. Classically, it is seen in otherwise healthy people but it does also occur in the immunocompromised. It is characterized by:
- a retinal and choroidal vasculitis;
- a necrotizing peripheral retinitis; and
- a severe vitritis.

The clinical disease may start insidiously, often with periorbital pain. There may be a mild anterior uveitis followed shortly afterwards by a decrease in visual acuity as the vitreous humour becomes cloudy and retinal necrosis begins (**Fig. 8.13**). The other eye may be involved in one-third of cases (usually within a few weeks) and up to 75% of patients develop retinal detachment.

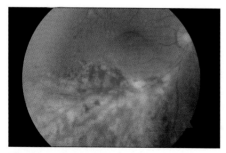

Fig. 8.11 *Haemorrhagic retinitis due to cytomegalovirus infection.*

Viruses and viral infections associated with retinitis

Herpes simplex virus type 1
Herpes simplex virus type 2
Cytomegalovirus
Epstein-Barr virus
Varicella-zoster virus
Rubella
Measles
Rift Valley fever

Fig. 8.12 *Viruses and viral infections associated with retinitis.*

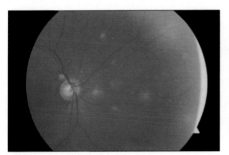

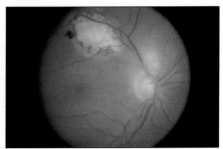

Fig. 8.13 *Acute retinial necrosis due to varicella-zoster virus infection.*

Fig. 8.14 *Scar following congenital toxoplasmal choroidoretinitis.*

Treatment is with high-dose intravenous aciclovir and systemic corticosteroids. Some authorities also recommend anticoagulation.

TOXOPLASMOSIS

The most common infection causing a posterior uveitis is toxoplasmosis. Although infection with *Toxoplasma gondii* is widespread, ocular disease is rare (involving 1–2% of those infected). Ocular toxoplasmosis usually represents reactivation of congenitally acquired infection (less than 1% of cases occur *de novo* in adults). In congenital cases, the disease reactivates around chorioretinal scars and presents in early adult life (**Fig. 8.14**). There is usually a vitritis with 'floaters' and decreased acuity. Pain and redness of the eye are rare.

The diagnosis is largely clinical, on the basis of symptoms and signs and the presence of an old scar. Serology is rarely helpful other than in establishing previous exposure. Recently, polymerase chain reaction analysis of samples of aqueous humour have been used to confirm the diagnosis.

Treatment is required in patients with visual loss and in immunocompromised patients. Small lesions may remit spontaneously. Systemic treatment is with sulphadiazine, pyrimethamine and corticosteroids.

TOXOCARIASIS

Infection with *Toxocara canis* larvae may occur in children and can cause a serious systemic illness known as visceral larva migrans. Ingestion of soil contaminated by dog and cat faeces is the probable portal of entry. Eye disease is extremely rare in visceral larva migrans. However, ocular toxocariasis also occurs in children and is rarely associated with systemic disease. It is almost always unilateral and presents with a decrease in visual acuity, sometimes with pain and redness in the eye. The pupil may appear white because of inflammation (leucocoria). The most common presentation is with an endophthalmitis, in which the vitreous humour is cloudy. There may be photophobia.

Sometimes in older children there is a macular chorioretinal granuloma with little inflammation in the vitreous humour. In older children and adults there may be peripheral granuloma formation with less severe effects on vision.

It is important to differentiate ocular toxocariasis from retinoblastoma; therefore investigations should include orbital computed tomography or magnetic resonance image scanning – calcification occurs in retinoblastomas but not in toxocariasis (**Fig. 8.15**).

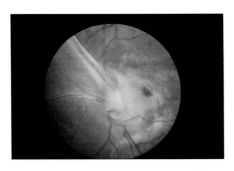

Fig. 8.15 *The fundus in ocular toxocariasis.*

Toxocara serology using an enzyme-linked immunosorbent assay to detect antibodies is helpful but eosinophilia is not a feature of ocular disease.

Treatment is disappointing although steroids may decrease inflammation and treatment may be required for retinal detachment. The role of specific antihelminthic agents is controversial.

OTHER OCULAR INFECTIONS

Other, miscellaneous infections of the eye are listed in **Figure 8.16.**

Miscellaneous infections that can affect the eyes

Bacteria	Condition caused
Mycobacterium leprae (leprosy)	eyelid inflammation keratitis iridocyclitis
Mycobacterium tuberculosis (TB)	iridocyclitis choroiditis optic neuritis
Borrelia burgdorferi (Lyme Disease)	choroiditis retinitis optic neuritis
Treponema pallidum (syphilis)	iridocyclitis choroiditis retinitis optic neuritis
Leptospira sp (leptospirosis)	iridocyclitis
Viruses	
Molluscum contagiosum	eyelid infection
Parasites	
Onchocerca volvulus (onchocerciasis)	keratitis choroiditis retinitis optic neuritis
Pediculosis capitis (lice)	eyelid infestation

Fig. 8.16 *Miscellaneous infections that can affect the eyes.*

ORBITAL CELLULITIS

In the preantibiotic era, cellulitis affecting the orbit was associated with significant mortality and loss of vision. Spread of infection from the nasal sinuses to the orbit is facilitated by the proximity of the sinuses to the orbit, the thin bones surrounding these structures and the presence of a valveless venous plexus. The danger of orbital cellulitis is that infection may spread to the central nervous system via the cavernous sinus. The usual organisms involved are those found in the sinuses: *H. influenzae* (rarer since the introduction of a vaccine), the pneumococcus and *S. aureus*.

Early symptoms and signs comprise redness and swelling of the eyelid in association with pain and cheimosis. As the infection progresses there is proptosis, restriction of eye movement and, in some cases, decreased visual acuity (**Figs 8.17** and **8.18**). Fever and headache are common. If there is ptosis, decreased corneal sensation or spread to the other eye, it is likely that the cavernous sinus is also involved.

The diagnosis is usually obvious but imaging (CT or MRI scanning) is required to assess proptosis, look for sinus disease and to detect periosteal involvement.

Treatment should involve emergency admission to hospital and the administration of intravenous antibiotics. Surgery may be required to drain a sinus or a subperiosteal abscess and the orbit may need to be decompressed if there is a rapid decrease in acuity.

PRESEPTAL CELLULITIS

This may mimic the early stages of orbital cellulitis with swelling and erythema of the lid but the subsequent signs of proptosis and disordered eye movements do not occur. This condition involves only the eyelid and is seen with infections in adjacent structures (e.g. the lacrimal gland) or following trauma (**Fig. 8.19**).

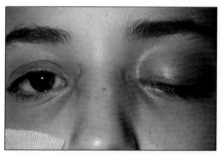

Fig. 8.17 *Orbital cellulitis following sinus infection.*

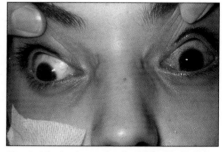

Fig. 8.18 *Ocular palsy in orbital cellulitis.*

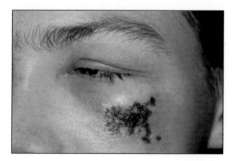

Fig. 8.19 *Preseptal cellulitis in association with primary cutaneous herpes simplex virus infection.*

chapter 9

Gastrointestinal Tract and Liver, Gall Bladder and Pancreas

When considering infections related to the alimentary system, it is most convenient to consider first those conditions relating to the luminal gastrointestinal tract and then those relating to the hepatobiliary system.

GASTROINTESTINAL TRACT

OESOPHAGUS

Infections limited to the oesophagus are unusual in immunocompetent people. In immunocompromised patients, the most common problem is oesophageal candidal infections (**Fig. 9.1**). This is a particular problem in patients infected with the human immunodeficiency virus (HIV) but it may occur in other patients taking corticosteroids, severely malnourished patients and those with T-lymphocyte defects not related to HIV.

Less commonly, the oesophagus may be affected by herpesvirus infection, either cytomegalovirus (CMV) or herpes simplex virus (HSV).

Oesophageal infections usually present with painful dysphagia. Candidal infections can cause widespread inflammation and ulceration; herpesvirus infections may be similar but can also lead to solitary ulcers or, sometimes, to a small number of discrete ulcers.

Infectious oesophagitis may be suspected clinically in susceptible patients with appropriate symptoms but it can be reliably diagnosed only with invasive investigations. Barium swallow confirms oesophagitis with or without ulceration but it cannot establish an aetiological diagnosis (**Fig. 9.2**). This can only be done by endoscopy. This may reveal obvious candidiasis but the cause of ulceration, if *Candida* is not obvious on direct vision, can only be determined by taking brushings and biopsies through the endoscope.

STOMACH

Helicobacter pylori infection

The normal low pH of the stomach lumen usually keeps the gastric mucosa and contents sterile. However, it is now established beyond reasonable doubt that infection of the

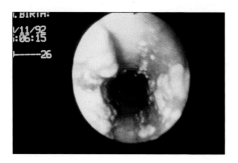

Fig. 9.1 *Endoscopic appearance of* Candida *in the oesophagus.*

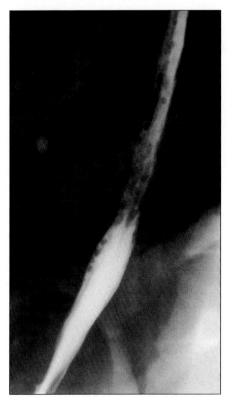

Fig. 9.2 *Barium swallow showing ulceration due to* Candida.

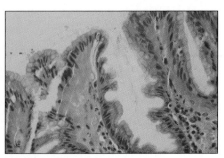

Fig. 9.3 *Gastric biopsy showing Helicobacter pylori.*

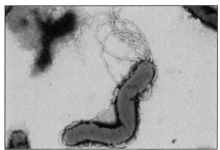

Fig. 9.4 *Electron micrograph showing Helicobacter pylori.*

mucosa by *H. pylori* occurs and is associated with gastritis, peptic ulcer disease and, possibly, gastric lymphoma. *H. pylori* is a small, spiral, Gram-negative bacillus that appears to inhabit the mucus layer overlying the gastric epithelial cells (Figs 9.3 and 9.4). It produces a potent urease, which, by producing ammonia, may help to neutralize gastric acid. The mechanism by which *H. pylori* produces gastric inflammation is not clear because the organism does not invade the mucosa. The inflammation might be immunologically mediated or it might come about through physicochemical alteration of gastric mucus, allowing gastric acid to damage epithelial cells.

The epidemiology of *H. pylori* infection has not been well worked out. Infections may be more common with age but they are also much more common in the tropics, with many children infected from an early age. The route of infection is unknown although it is often presumed to be the faecal–oral route.

Treatment to eradicate *H. pylori* infection reduces the incidence of gastritis and duodenal ulcer. When triple therapy– a proton pump inhibitor (e.g. omeprazole), metronidazole and clarithromycin – is used, ulcer healing is as good as with histamine-2 antagonists (80–90%) with a much lower relapse rate.

Other gastric infections

Like any other part of the gastrointestinal tract, the stomach can be affected by CMV infection in immunocompromised hosts. This usually causes multiple small mucosal ulcers. The main clinical problems are usually epigastric pain or gastrointestinal blood loss, or both.

Tuberculosis can occur in the stomach and may mimic an ulcer or be clinically occult. Infection may arise from haemotogenous spread but often, particularly in the past, it arises in patients with active pulmonary tuberculosis who have swallowed infectious sputum.

ENTERIC INFECTIONS

GASTROENTERITIS

Gastric acid helps to maintain the sterility of the stomach contents, and normal intestinal motility ensures a normal distribution and flow of bowel flora. Anaerobic bacteria make up 99% of the bowel flora. Further protection against gastrointestinal infection comes from lymphoid tissue in Peyer's patches and from secretory immunoglobulin (Ig) A on the mucosal surface.

Micro-organisms may cause disease in the gastrointestinal tract either by:
* adhering to or invading enterocytes (or both); or
* by producing bacterial products, such as enterotoxins, that can cause mucosal damage or increase net intestinal secretions.

Most enteric infections present as gastroenteritis with diarrhoea or vomiting or both. The type of symptoms and the localization of the infection in the gastrointestinal tract depend on the infecting organism. Worldwide, gastroenteritis accounts for more morbidity and mortality, especially in children in the tropics, than almost any other condition. Diarrhoea results from infections when the absorptive capacity of the gastrointestinal tract is overwhelmed. Vomiting may accompany diarrhoea, especially when the diarrhoea is of small bowel origin, or it may occur as an isolated feature.

There are three main mechanisms by which infective diarrhoea can arise:
* noninflammatory diarrhoea usually results from the action of bacterial enterotoxins and predominantly affects the stomach and small bowel;
* inflammatory diarrhoea results from bacterial invasion and the elaboration of cytotoxins and usually involves the large bowel; and
* penetrating infections, for which the distal small bowel is the usual site of invasion and in which there are usually significant systemic symptoms.

NONINFLAMMATORY DIARRHOEA

Viral infections are a common cause of diarrhoea, particularly in children. Rotavirus is one of the most common causes, leading to vomiting, abdominal distension, diarrhoea and fever (Fig. 9.5). Other viruses, such as Norwalk agent, astrovirus and other small round-structured viruses, can produce a similar clinical picture. The pathogenesis of viral gastroenteritis is not entirely clear but it probably involves subtle damage to absorptive cells in the small intestinal villi. These viruses are spread easily from patient to patient by aerosol, and so outbreaks in nurseries and hospital wards are not uncommon.

The classic bacterial cause of noninflammatory, or secretory, diarrhoea is *Vibrio cholerae*. Cholera is endemic in many parts of the tropics and epidemics occur regularly. The disease is spread by the faecal–oral route and is associated with poor sanitation and overcrowding. Cholera toxin binds to enterocytes via the B subunit of the toxin and the A

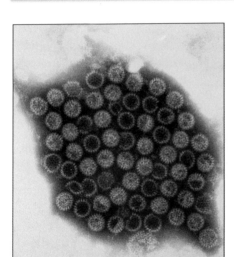

Fig. 9.5 *Electron micrograph of rotavirus.*

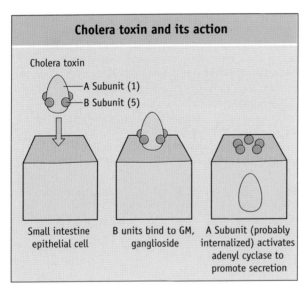

Fig. 9.6 *Cholera toxin and its action.*

subunit activates adenyl cyclase in the intestinal mucosal cells (**Fig. 9.6**). Levels of intracellular cyclic adenosine monophosphate rise, inhibiting sodium–chloride-linked absorption. This results in a net flow of chloride ions and water into the gut lumen.

Patients with cholera develop severe, watery diarrhoea, sometimes described as 'rice water stools', and they can rapidly become dehydrated (**Fig. 9.7**). Oral, and sometimes intravenous, rehydration therapy is vitally important and tetracycline therapy can eradicate the cholera bacteria. The old parenteral vaccine is largely ineffective for prophylaxis, but newer, oral vaccines look promising.

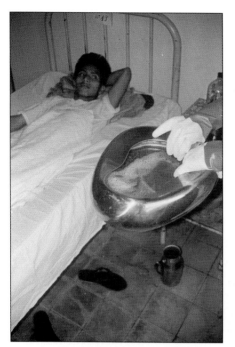

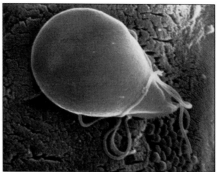

Fig. 9.8 *Transmission electron micrograph of* Giardia lamblia.

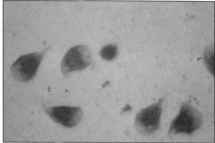

Fig. 9.7 *Patient with cholera in Peru.*

Fig. 9.9 Giardia lamblia *trophozoites in stool sample.*

Other bacteria also produce gastroenteritis via the production of toxins. Food poisoning due to *Staphylococcus aureus* or *Bacillus cereus* occurs when toxin is ingested after it has been preformed in the food by multiplying bacteria. Most other organisms, such as *Escherichia coli*, *V. cholerae*, *Clostridium perfringens* and, sometimes, *B. cereus* multiply within the gut lumen and elaborate their toxins in the intestine.

Parasites, such as *Giardia lamblia*, *Cryptosporidium parvum* and *Isospora belli*, may produce acute noninflammatory diarrhoea, especially in children (**Figs 9.8** and **9.9**). They can also lead to chronic problems, particularly in HIV-positive patients.

Chronic noninflammatory diarrhoea

Some infections may lead to a more chronic diarrhoea of small bowel origin. All acute infections, notably rotavirus infections and giardiasis, may lead to damage to brush border enzymes and a secondary lactase deficiency. The inability to digest lactose adequately leads to diarrhoea from the osmotic effects of lactose in the lumen.

Bacterial overgrowth in the small intestine may also lead to chronic diarrhoea. This is usually associated with some form of pre-existing bowel problem such as diverticula, blind loops following surgery or impaired small intestinal motility (e.g. with diabetes mellitus or scleroderma) (**Fig. 9.10**).

Tropical sprue is a condition sometimes described in people from nontropical areas who have spent prolonged periods in the tropics. Diarrhoea is often accompanied by malabsorption. The aetiology is obscure but may be related to bacterial overgrowth, for it often responds to prolonged antibiotic therapy.

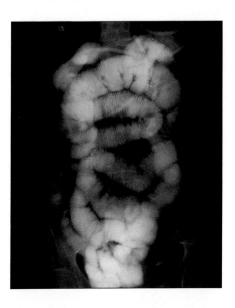

Fig. 9.10 *Barium follow-through study showing stasis in scleroderma – a risk for bacterial overgrowth.*

Fig. 9.11 *Infections that may present with dysentery (bloody diarrhoea).*

Infections that may present with bloody diarrhoea	
Bacteria	**Parasites**
Salmonella spp.	*Entamoeba histolytica*
Shigella spp.	*Schistosoma mansoni*
Campylobacter jejuni	*Schistosoma japonicum*
Vibrio parahaemolyticus	*Balantidium coli*
Clostridium difficile	*Trichinella spiralis*
Clostridium perfringens	*Plasmodium falciparum*
Enterohaemorrhagic *Escherichia coli*	

INFLAMMATORY DIARRHOEA

Acute inflammatory diarrhoea is usually bacterial in origin, although some parasites produce dysenteric syndromes. The main causes are shown in **Figure 9.11**. Usually both the small and large intestine are involved and the inflammation commonly leads to the presence of pus cells in the stool.

These infections usually present as acute dysentery with mild fever, abdominal pain and diarrhoea. Vomiting can sometimes also be a feature. Blood and mucus usually appears in the stool and microscopy shows red cells and polymorphs (**Fig. 9.12**). Sigmoidoscopy may show an inflamed rectal mucosa, sometimes with ulceration (**Fig. 9.13**). Occasionally, especially in the case of infections with *Salmonella* spp. and *Campylobacter* spp., patients may become toxic and very unwell, with some developing toxic megacolon and its attendant risk of perforation (**Fig. 9.14**).

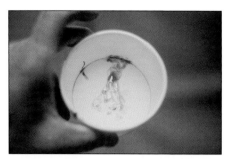

Fig. 9.12 *Macroscopic appearance of the stool in bacillary dysentery.*

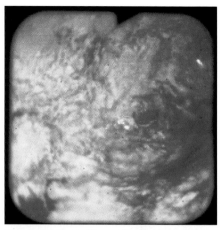

Fig. 9.13 *Sigmoidoscopic appearance of colitis caused by infection.*

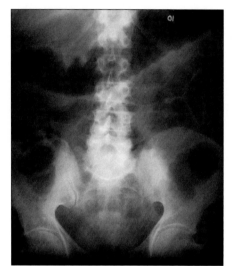

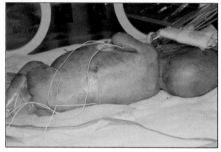

Fig. 9.15 *Infant with necrotizing enterocolitis and distended abdomen.*

Fig. 9.14 *Plain abdominal X-ray showing toxic dilatation in* Salmonella *infection.*

Necrotizing enterocolitis

This can be a serious condition in infants, particularly low-birth-weight babies (Fig. 9.15). A variety of Gram-negative Enterobacteriaceae and anaerobic bacteria have been implicated in nectrotizing enterocolitis. There is severe inflammation of the bowel and a high risk of perforation. The children have fever, abdominal distension and bloody diarrhoea and they may have apnoeic spells.

Pig-bel

Pig-bel, a condition described in both children and adults in Papua New Guinea, presents with severe abdominal pain, vomiting and bloody diarrhoea. It may proceed rapidly to septic shock. It is probably due to infection with *C. perfringens* type C, the bacterial toxins (a and b) of which lead to a necrotizing enteritis (Fig. 9.16).

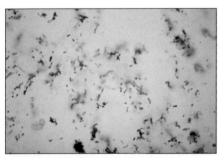

Fig. 9.16 *Section of small bowel infiltrated with* Clostridium perfringens *in pig-bel.*

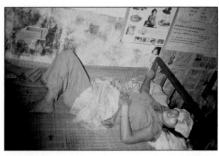

Fig. 9.17 *Typical appearance of a patient with typhoid. Note the apathetic facies.*

Fig. 9.18 *Perforation of the small bowel in typhoid.*

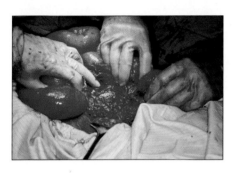

Chronic inflammatory diarrhoea

Some organisms lead to chronic inflammation in the gastrointestinal tract, which may present with chronic diarrhoea with or without abdominal pain. Tuberculosis may present this way. Recurrent or relapsing intestinal amoebiasis can also cause chronic diarrhoea, as can fungi such as *Histoplasma capsulatum* and *Paracoccidioides brasiliensis*. Infection with *Yersinia* spp. and *Entamoeba histolytica* can cause chronic inflammation in the ileocaecum, mimicking Crohn's disease.

Invasive gastrointestinal infections

Some infectious agents penetrate the gastrointestinal tract, causing systemic features that usually obscure the gastrointestinal symptoms. This often takes the form of enteric fever.

TYPHOID

Salmonella typhi leads to typhoid, the classic enteric fever. Spread by the faecal oral route, with humans as the only host, this Gram-negative rod penetrates the intestinal mucosa and multiplies in Peyer's patches. The bacilli then disseminate via blood and lymphatic vessels. There follows a sustained bacteraemia and the risk of distant seeding. Usually the main problem is fever in a listless patient (**Fig. 9.17**). Headache and a dry cough are common symptoms. Splenomegaly and rose spots are signs that appear in fewer than 25% of cases. Gastrointestinal symptoms are not a major feature although diarrhoea occurs. There may be late complications, such as intestinal haemorrhage from small intestinal ulcers, and bowel perforation (**Fig. 9.18**).

Fig. 9.19 *Causes of enteric fever syndrome.*

Causes of enteric fever syndrome
Salmonella typhi *Salmonella paratyphi* A and B *Campylobacter fetus* *Yersinia enterocolitica* *Yersinia pseudotuberculosis*

Fig. 9.19 *Causes of enteric fever syndrome.*

The diagnosis is usually made by blood culture, although culture of bone marrow is more sensitive. Stool cultures and rectal swabs are useful in developing countries where blood culture is difficult. Treatment is with antibiotics appropriate to the local resistance patterns. Many strains of *Salmonella typhi* are multi-resistant but fluoroquinolones remain the treatment of choice. Rarely, some people become chronic carriers and excretors of *S. typhi*. These people usually have some form of gallbladder disease, often gallstones. Eradication of carriage may be achieved by prolonged quinolone treatment but sometimes cholecystectomy is used.

OTHER CAUSES OF ENTERIC FEVER

A variety of bacteria may cause an enteric fever syndrome (**Fig. 9.19**). Infections with *Yersinia* spp. are associated with iron overload and are seen in patients with serious medical conditions, such as chronic liver disease. Infections with both *Yersinia* spp. and *Campylobacter fetus* may present with septic arthritis. *Yersinia* may cause ileocaecal inflammation mimicking appendicitis and, in children, it may be a cause of mesenteric adenitis.

OTHER GASTROINTESTINAL INFECTIONS

PARASITES

Many helminth infections invade the gut as part of their life cycles. They may cause abdominal symptoms and there is usually an associated eosinophilia. *Strongyloides stercoralis* may cause abdominal discomfort as well as diarrhoea (**Fig. 9.20**). This important worm has a complicated life cycle and can persist through autoinfection. This persistence carries a risk of dissemination, which leads to a severe hyperinfection syndrome in patients who become immunosuppressed. Other nematodes, such as *Ascaris lumbricoides* and *Ancylostoma duodenale* may cause abdominal pain and distension (**Fig. 9.21**).

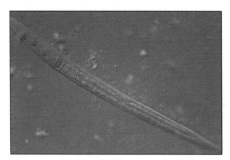

Fig. 9.20 Strongyloides stercoralis *larva in stool.*

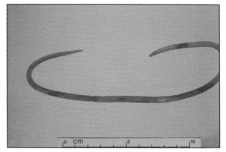

Fig. 9.21 Ascaris lumbricoides *(adult worm).*

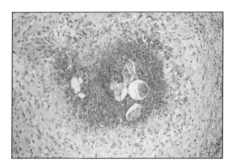

Fig. 9.22 *Rectal biopsy showing* Schistosoma mansoni *egg inside a granuloma.*

Schistosoma mansoni may present with intestinal symptoms such as diarrhoea (**Fig. 9.22**). The majority of infections, however, are asymptomatic. Cestode (tapeworm) infections rarely cause symptoms although patients may notice the passage of worm segments in the stool.

Trypanosoma cruzi, the cause of Chagas' disease, can damage the myenteric plexus. The usual manifestation of this is achalasia, and patients may present with megaoesophagus and recurrent chest infections from overspill (**Fig. 9.23**). The colon can also be affected, leading to chronic constipation and a dilated colon, analogous to the situation in Hirschsprung's disease.

Whipple's disease

This is a chronic, systemic disease that primarily affects males. Most of the morbidity arises from the gastrointestinal manifestations of diarrhoea, malabsorption and weight loss. Arthralgia and occasional fevers are also common features. Small bowel biopsy reveals macrophages stuffed with period acid–Schiff-positive organisms that have recently been identified and named *Tropheryma whippeli* (**Fig. 9.24**). Treatment is with a prolonged course of oral co-trimoxazole after initial treatment with parenteral penicillin and streptomycin.

Abdominal tuberculosis

Tuberculosis can affect any part of the gastrointestinal tract. Although *Mycobacterium bovis* used to be a common cause, most cases today are due to *Mycobacterium tuberculosis*. The organism may reach the abdomen by direct spread from the chest, haematogenous or lymphatic spread or by swallowing infectious sputum. In the intestine, the terminal ileum and caecum are the most common sites of infection. Patients may present with a right iliac fossa mass or with symptoms of subacute small bowel obstruction (**Figs 9.25** and **9.26**). Iron deficiency secondary to chronic blood loss is common, but frank bleeding or perforation are rare. Occasionally, if there is extensive small bowel involvement, malabsorption is the presenting feature. Intestinal tuberculosis can be difficult to distinguish from Crohn's disease (**Fig. 9.27**). Nonspecific symptoms such as malaise, weight loss and fever are common and may be the only symptoms.

Tuberculosis may also present as chronic peritonitis with abdominal distension secondary to ascites. There may be systemic symptoms of tuberculosis. In addition to ascites, there may be marked inflammation and induration of the omentum and peritoneum, leading to a 'doughy' feel when the abdomen is palpated.

Abdominal lymph nodes may be affected by tuberculosis and may be the first presenting feature, either if they are palpable or if they are found incidentally when imaging is performed on patients with unexplained fever.

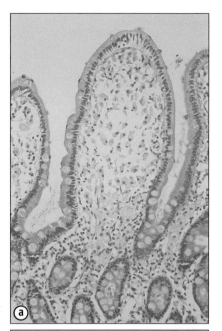

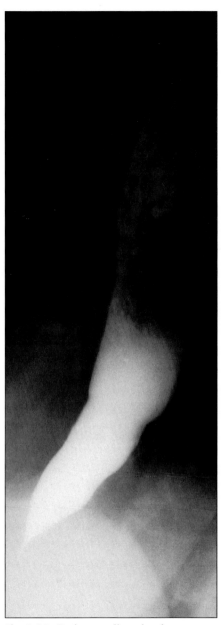

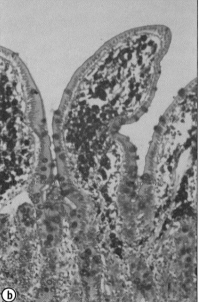

Fig. 9.23 *Barium swallow showing achalasia, a late feature of Chagas' disease.*

Fig. 9.24 *Whipple's disease: (a) small bowel biopsy in Whipple's disease showing 'foamy' macrophages in the villi; (b) small bowel biopsy with periodic acid–Schiff–positive bacteria in macrophages.*

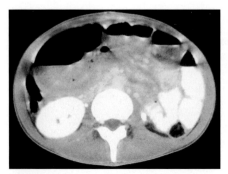

Fig. 9.25 *CT scan showing thickened, matted bowel in tuberculosis.*

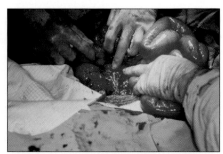

Fig. 9.26 *Intestinal tuberculosis at laparotomy with tubercles on the bowel surface.*

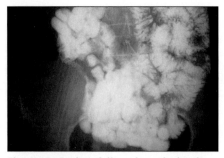

Fig. 9.27 *Barium follow-through showing abnormal terminal ileum in intestinal tuberculosis.*

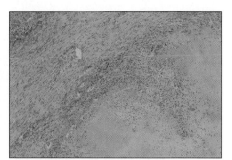

Fig. 9.28 *Biopsy showing typical tuberculous granulomas.*

Both intestinal and peritoneal tuberculosis may be associated with infected intra-abdominal nodes.

Imaging the abdomen with contrast studies or computed tomography (CT) scans may show indirect evidence of tuberculosis. Definitive diagnosis can only be achieved by obtaining tissue for histology and culture (**Fig. 9.28**). This might be possible laparoscopically or by limited laparotomy. Emergency laparotomy may be required for acute obstruction. Culture of ascites or peritoneal biopsies is important because acid-fast bacilli are rarely seen on microscopy of ascites. Treatment is by conventional antituberculous chemotherapy.

Antibiotic-associated diarrhoea

The normal gut flora may be affected by the administration of broad-spectrum antibiotics. This alteration in bacterial flora may lead to diarrhoea, usually by promoting the growth of *Clostridium difficile*, a Gram-positive, spore-forming bacillus. This organism causes a colitis by elaborating potent enterotoxins. Enterotoxin A is probably the principal cause of colonic inflammation. Affected patients present with diarrhoea and may have systemic upset, such as fever and tachycardia. Severely affected patients may develop a pancolitis and may even go on to develop a toxic megacolon.

The disease should be suspected in patients who develop diarrhoea during or after antibiotic therapy, particularly if they are in hospital. Sigmoidoscopy may reveal a mild proctitis and more florid cases sometimes have a pseudomembranous colitis with yellow–white plaques of membrane that are adherent to the colonic mucosa (**Fig. 9.29**).

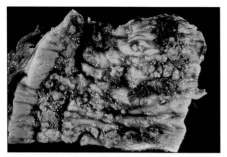

Fig. 9.29 *Post-mortem specimen of bowel showing pseudomembranous colitis.*

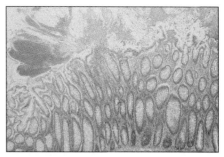

Fig. 9.30 *Histology showing pseudomembrane in* Clostridium difficile *colitis (haematoxylin and eosin stain).*

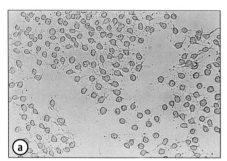

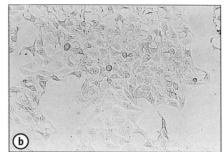

Fig. 9.31 *(a) Cytopathic effect of* Clostridium difficile *toxin on Vero cell culture. (b) control.*

This can be confirmed by biopsy (**Fig. 9.30**). Diagnosis is by demonstration of the C. *difficile* toxin in the stool. Although toxin A is probably most important pathophysiologically, toxin B is the product that is detected by diagnostic tests. It is cytotoxic to Vero cells in tissue culture, so this is a common detection system used in laboratories (**Fig. 9.31**). More recently, reliable enzyme-linked immunosorbent assays have become available. Culture of C. *difficile* is not, of itself, sufficient for a diagnosis of antibiotic-associated diarrhoea because up to 3% of people carry C. *difficile* in their stools. C. *difficile* may be responsible for nosocomial outbreaks of diarrhoea because its spores are hardy and may spread throughout hospital wards.

Treatment is aimed at stopping any antibiotic therapy (if possible) and maintaining adequate hydration. Oral metronidazole and oral vancomycin are equally effective at eradicating C. *difficile* from the gastrointestinal tract and should be given for 7 days. Relapses are not uncommon, particularly in debilitated hospital patients.

Travellers' diarrhoea

Many people will experience diarrhoea and vomiting when travelling abroad, especially to the tropics. This may be because travellers are exposed to new pathogens to which they have no immunity or because the risk of ingesting contaminated food and drink is higher in developing countries. A wide variety of organisms may cause travellers' diarrhoea (**Fig. 9.32**). Most cases settle spontaneously with conservative rehydration therapy. Antibiotic therapy with a quinolone antibiotic may shorten the duration of symptoms but is rarely justified.

Common causes of travellers' diarrhoea

Enterotoxigenic *Escherichia coli*
Enteroadherent *Escherichia coli*
Shigella spp.
Salmonella spp.
Campylobacter spp.
Aeromonas spp.
Rotavirus
Giardia lamblia
Entamoeba histolytica
Cryptosporidium parvum

Fig. 9.32 *Common causes of travellers' diarrhoea. Note that no pathogen is identified in almost half of all cases.*

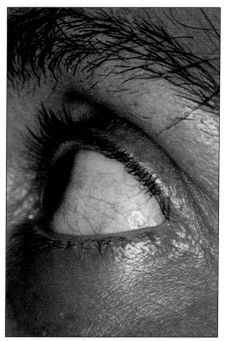

Fig. 9.33 *Jaundice in hepatitis A virus infection.*

Also, antibiotic prophylaxis with drugs such as doxycycline or ciprofloxacin can reduce the risk of travellers' diarrhoea but, again, the widespread use of such prophylaxis should be avoided in order to minimize costs and reduce the risk of antibiotic resistance.

HEPATOBILIARY SYSTEM

HEPATITIS

Infective hepatitis can be caused by a variety of agents, most of which are viruses. Generally, they all cause inflammation of the liver which may be mild but can be very severe and lead to acute liver failure as a result of massive hepatic necrosis. In addition, some of these hepatitis viruses, notably hepatitis B virus, may persist and cause chronic hepatic inflammation, leading to chronic liver disease.

Hepatitis A virus

Hepatitis A virus (HAV) is a ribonucleic acid (RNA) virus that is transmitted by the faecal–oral route and is common worldwide. It usually causes sporadic cases of hepatitis but it may be associated with outbreaks, often from a common food source. The incubation period ranges from 2–6 weeks. Many children under the age of 8 years have asymptomatic infections whereas adults usually have a prodrome of mild fever, malaise and nausea followed by jaundice (**Fig. 9.33**). Fulminant hepatitis is very rare. Occasionally patients with HAV infection develop prolonged cholestatic jaundice. This may be improved by a short course of corticosteroids. Otherwise treatment is symptomatic and recovery leads to life-long immunity.

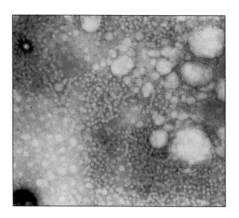

Fig. 9.34 *Electron micrograph of hepatitis B virus particles.*

Infection with HAV infection is diagnosed by finding anti-hepatitis A IgM in the serum. Close contacts of the patients may be offered gammaglobulin and, nowadays, immunization to prevent secondary cases. Travellers to areas of the world where HAV infection is common can be offered either human immunoglobulin as passive immunization or HAV vaccine for longer-lasting active immunization.

Hepatitis B virus

Hepatitis B virus (HBV) is the most important hepatitis virus because of its infectivity and its ability to cause chronic liver disease and hepatocellular carcinoma. It is a deoxyribonucleic acid (DNA) virus (**Fig. 9.34**) that is spread parenterally, usually by contaminated blood or needles, by sexual intercourse or from mother to child. In some areas of the world, such as China and sub-Saharan Africa, vertical transmission is extremely common. Nosocomial transmission has been a considerable problem, particularly in haemodialysis units.

The incubation period ranges from 6 weeks to 6 months. Many infections are subclinical with only about 25% of infected adults developing jaundice. Rarely, an immune complex disease occurs, with arthralgia, skin rash and fever. Fulminant hepatitis, though more common than in HAV infection, is still rare.

Although 95% of infections are cleared, the remaining 5% of patients are chronically infected. Some of these develop chronic active hepatitis with a consequent risk of cirrhosis, liver failure and hepatocellular carcinoma.

Serological diagnosis is essential in HBV infections and there are a variety of markers that can be clinically helpful (**Fig. 9.35**). In the initial stages of infection, HBV surface antigen (HBsAg) appears. This denotes infectivity. Early on about 15% of patients will be HBsAg negative but will have IgM antibodies against HBV core antigen (anti-HBc). As clinical recovery occurs, HBsAg disappears and anti-HBc IgG increases. The appearance of anti-HBs (anti-HBsAg IgG) implies protective immunity. In contrast, HBV 'e' antigen (HBeAg) positivity implies high infectivity and is associated with chronic infection.

Although most people clear their infection with HBV, those who fail to clear it risk morbidity and death from liver disease. Interferon therapy can, in selected patients, promote clearance of the virus and a return to normal liver histology and function. Trials with newer antiviral agents are in progress.

Good recombinant vaccines are available for active immunization of those at risk of HBV infection, such as health-care workers. For those exposed to HBV through needle-stick injuries or close contacts with patients with acute HBV infection, an accelerated vaccine course in conjunction with human hyperimmune globulin can be offered.

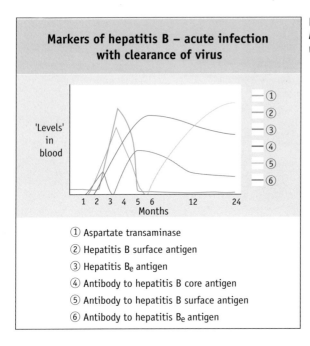

Fig. 9.35 *Markers of hepatitis B – acute infection with clearance of virus.*

Markers of hepatitis B – acute infection with clearance of virus

'Levels' in blood

Months

① Aspartate transaminase
② Hepatitis B surface antigen
③ Hepatitis B$_e$ antigen
④ Antibody to hepatitis B core antigen
⑤ Antibody to hepatitis B surface antigen
⑥ Antibody to hepatitis B$_e$ antigen

Delta virus

This is a defective RNA virus that is transmissible but requires the presence of HBV to replicate in human hepatocytes. It is seen as a superinfection in patients with chronic HBV infection, most commonly in intravenous drug users. Co-infection with delta virus increases the risk of fulminant hepatitis in acute infections, and superinfection increases the risk of progression in those with chronic liver disease. Delta virus can be detected by antibody tests and by molecular techniques. There is no vaccine, although if hepatitis B vaccination is given to prevent HBV infection, delta virus infection cannot occur.

Non-A, non-B hepatitis

After HAV and HBV were recognized, it became clear that there were cases of viral hepatitis, particularly following blood transfusion, that could not be explained. Many of these cases are now known to be due to hepatitis C virus (HCV), an RNA flavivirus. In addition to transfusion recipients, intravenous drug users are commonly infected. Sexual transmission occurs but is relatively uncommon. Many cases of HCV infection have no exposure history. The natural history of HCV infection is far from clear but most patients have subclinical infection. Some progress to chronic liver disease, cirrhosis and, occasionally, hepatocellular carcinoma. Infection with HCV has been associated with cryoglobulinaemia and may present as a vasculitis (**Fig. 9.36**).

Hepatitis C virus infection can be diagnosed by anti-HCV antibody detection or by finding HCV RNA in blood using the polymerase chain reaction. Interferon therapy can lead to improvement in liver function and histology but relapse after stopping treatment is common. The long-term benefits of interferon are not known.

In addition to HCV, at least three other hepatitis viruses have been found recently. Hepatitis E virus (HEV) appears to be spread enterally and is responsible for some epidemics of hepatitis in Asia. Pregnant women seem to be at risk of fulminant hepatitis when infected with this virus. Hepatitis F virus (HFV) infections and hepatitis G virus

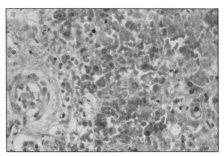

Fig. 9.37 *Histological appearance of hepatitis due to herpes simplex virus (haematoxylin and eosin stain).*

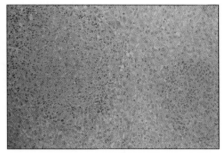

Fig. 9.38 *Hepatic granuloma caused by Q fever (haematoxylin and eosin stain).*

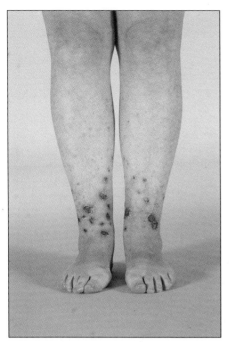

Fig. 9.36 *Vasculitis in hepatitis C virus infection.*

(HGV) infections are spread parenterally. Infections with HEV can be detected serologically but tests for HFV and HGV are still at the research stage.

Other viruses that cause hepatitis

Herpesviruses sometimes cause hepatitis in acute primary infections. Epstein–Barr virus and cytomegalovirus do this more commonly than herpes simplex virus (**Fig. 9.37**) or varicella–zoster virus (VZV). In immunocompetent patients, the hepatitis is self-limiting but fulminant disease can occur in immunocompromised patients, particularly after bone marrow transplantation. Chronic liver disease does not occur after herpesvirus infections.

Granulomatous hepatitis

A wide variety of infections and noninfective conditions may lead to inflammation in the liver and the formation of giant cell granulomas (**Fig. 9.38**). The infective causes are listed in **Figure 9.39**. The hepatitis improves with treatment of the underlying cause and, in many cases, is self-limiting.

LIVER ABSCESS

Micro-organisms frequently pass to the liver either through the systemic circulation or the portal venous system and may cause abscesses.

Pyogenic liver abscess

Most abscesses are caused by Gram-negative bacilli, both aerobic and anaerobic, and the majority occur as a result of biliary sepsis. However, Gram-positive organisms are also found, particularly *Streptococcus milleri*. Enterococcal infections are seen in association with biliary tree manipulations, such as stenting. Some liver abscesses arise from gastrointestinal infections causing portal pyaemia or from seeding during a systemic bacteraemia (**Fig. 9.40**). Liver abscesses were seen as common complications of appendicitis in the preantibiotic era. Now, patients with pyogenic liver abscess are older (middle-aged to elderly) and the sources of infection include diverticular disease, inflammatory bowel disease and malignancy.

The symptoms are often nonspecific but right upper quadrant discomfort and shoulder tip pain occur if the liver capsule is stretched. Fever is commonly but not invariably present. A neutrophil leucocytosis and abnormal liver function tests are helpful but not always seen.

Diagnosis is usually made by imaging; ultrasound being the investigation of choice. CT scanning (**Fig. 9.41**) and MRI scanning are also useful.

Treatment consists of a drainage procedure in conjunction with appropriate antibiotic therapy. Open surgical drainage, once common, is now being replaced by ultrasound or CT-guided aspiration and drainage. Therapy can be monitored by repeated ultrasound imaging.

Amoebic liver abscess

Intestinal infection with *Entamoeba histolytica* may lead to trophozoites entering the portal venous system and arriving in the liver, where they cause abscess formation. Half the patients with amoebic liver abscesses give no history of amoebic dysentery and have no

Infective causes of hepatic granuloma
Mycobacteria
Brucella spp.
Coxiella burnetii (Q fever)
Francisella tularensis (tularaemia)
Treponema pallidum (secondary syphilis)
Histoplasma capsulatum
Coccidioides imitis
Cytomegalovirus
Epstein–Barr virus

Fig. 9.39 *Infective causes of hepatic granuloma.*

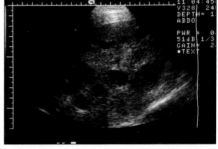

Fig. 9.40 *Ultrasound of pyogenic liver abscesses.*

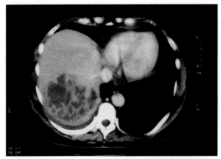

Fig. 9.41 *CT scan of a loculated liver abscess caused by* **Streptococcus milleri.**

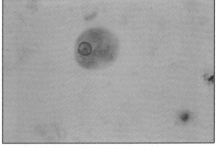

Fig. 9.42 *Cysts of* Entamoeba histolytica *in stool.*

evidence of amoebae in the stool (**Fig. 9.42**). Amoebic liver abscesses usually present with fever and hepatic pain and tenderness. There may be an elevated right hemidiaphragm on the chest X-ray (**Fig. 9.43**).

Diagnosis is by ultrasound or other imaging. Unlike pyogenic abscesses, amoebic abscesses are much more likely to be single (**Fig. 9.44**). In endemic areas, where amoebiasis is common, such an abscess may be treated empirically with metronidazole but if there are doubts or if pain is marked, the abscess should be aspirated. The material aspirated, sometimes said to resemble anchovy sauce, consists mainly of necrotic liver and therefore pus cells and amoebae are rarely seen on microscopy. Most patients have positive serological tests for *E. histolytica*. Rarely, amoebic abscesses may rupture through the diaphragm into the right pleural space or into the pericardium.

With or without drainage, the amoebic abscess can be treated with metronidazole for 10 days, followed by diloxanide furoate to eliminate any intestinal cysts.

Hydatid cysts

Humans sometimes become secondary hosts for the dog tapeworm, *Echinococcus granulosus* (see **Fig 15.32**). Eggs from dog faeces can be ingested, enter the intestine and pass into the circulation and then be deposited in a variety of organs, most commonly the liver. The tissue cysts have an internal capsule, which is a germinal layer from which brood capsules, or 'daughter cysts', containing infective scolices protrude (**Fig. 9.45**). This complex structure is sometimes a useful clue to the diagnosis when ultrasound (**Fig. 9.46**) or

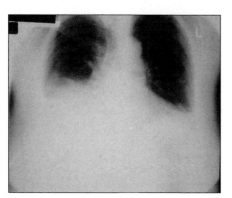

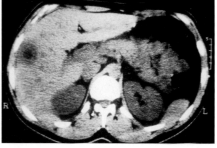

Fig. 9.44 *CT scan of the liver showing an amoebic liver abscess.*

Fig. 9.43 *Chest X-ray showing elevated right diaphragm in patient with liver abscess.*

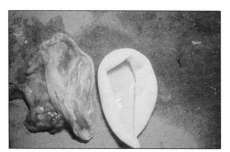

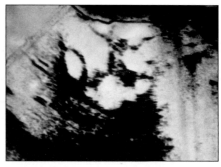

Fig. 9.45 *Operative specimen showing daughter cysts in hydatid cyst.*

Fig. 9.46 *Liver ultrasound showing hydatid cysts.*

CT scanning (**Fig. 9.47**) is performed. Many hydatid cysts are asymptomatic and may be discovered incidentally. Sometimes, depending on the target organ, symptoms arise as a result of pressure from the expanding cyst (**Fig. 9.48**). In the liver, this may cause pain as the liver capsule is stretched or jaundice may arise from biliary tract compression.

Diagnosis is by imaging and by positive serology. Eosinophilia is present in only about 25% of cases. Aspiration of cysts is contraindicated as there is a high risk of rupture and further spread of infective scolices. Open surgical removal remains the treatment of choice. Antihelminthic treatment options are limited but there is increasing evidence that the combination of albendazole and praziquantel is useful. These drugs may be given before surgery to reduce the risk of spillage of viable scolices, and they may be given in inoperable cases.

A similar but more aggressive condition is caused by *Echinococcus multilocularis,* a canine tapeworm found in wolves in Siberia. The cysts are not well encapsulated and tend to spread through the liver and other affected organs.

GALLBLADDER

Cholecystitis

The presence of gallstones in the gallbladder may lead to acute inflammation of the gallbladder (**Figs 9.49** and **9.50**). The mechanism of the inflammation is complex and

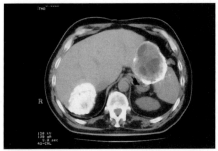

Fig. 9.47 CT scan of the liver showing hydatid cysts.

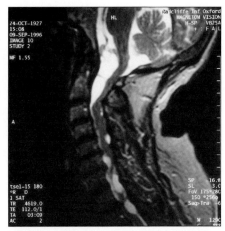

Fig. 9.48 MRI scan showing hydatid cysts compressing the cervical cord.

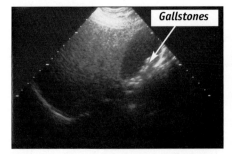

Fig. 9.49 Ultrasound showing gallstones.

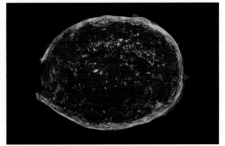

Fig. 9.50 Gross specimen of gall bladder showing acute cholecystitis.

involves blockage of the cystic duct by one or more stones, gallbladder distension and compromise to the blood supply and lymphatic drainage. Infection may then ensue.

Acute cholecystitis is usually associated with upper abdominal pain, which later localizes to the right upper quadrant. There is associated nausea and vomiting. There may be peritonism, and pain in the right shoulder tip is sometimes present. There is often a moderate fever and slight jaundice. Many patients' symptoms resolve over a few days but about one-third develop complications.

Diagnosis is usually clinical, aided by ultrasonography, which demonstrates stones in the gallbladder and may show a dilated gallbladder or fluid around the gallbladder. Infection is usually due to bowel flora, mainly Enterobacteriaceae (e.g. *E. coli*, *Klebsiella* spp.) and anaerobes.

Treatment of acute attacks involves appropriate symptomatic therapy for pain and vomiting. Antibiotics are usually given (generally a combination of a cephalosporin and an aminoglycoside) but have not been shown to affect clinical outcome.

Complications of cholecystitis include acute gangrene and perforation of the gallbladder, empyema of the gallbladder and pancreatitis (**Fig. 9.51**). Surgery is usually required for these complications, as are perioperative antibiotics. The role of surgery for uncomplicated acute cholecystitis is controversial. Traditionally, surgery has been delayed until the acute phase settles but 'hot' surgery is increasingly being performed at the time of the acute presentation.

Cholangitis

This term implies inflammation or infection of the hepatic and common bile ducts. There is probably always some cholangitis in association with acute cholecystitis. More severe cholangitis occurs, however, in the setting of common bile duct obstruction by stones or tumours (**Fig. 9.52**). Ascending cholangitis may also occur with pancreatitis or following endoscopic retrograde cholangiopancreatography (ERCP). Patients often have Charcot's triad of fever, rigors and jaundice. There is usually pain in the right upper quadrant of the abdomen.

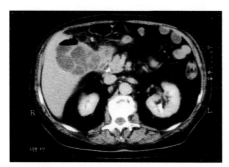

Fig. 9.51 *CT scan of empyema of the gallbladder.*

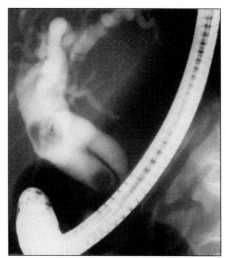

Fig. 9.52 *Gallstones in the common bile duct demonstrated by endoscopic retrograde cholangiopancreatography.*

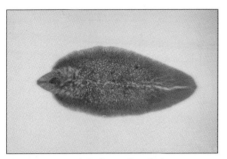

Fig. 9.53 Fasciola hepatica *fluke.*

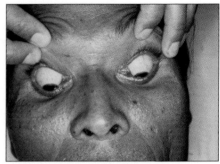

Fig. 9.54 *Jaundice resulting from* **Clonorchis sinensis** *flukes obstructing bile duct.*

Unlike the situation with acute cholecystitis, many patients with cholangitis are bacteraemic, usually with Gram-negative bacilli and anaerobes. Laboratory tests are nonspecific but a leucocytosis and deranged liver function tests are common. Ultrasound may show a dilated biliary tree (not an invariable feature) and ERCP may provide a more detailed assessment of the ducts.

Treatment consists of parenteral antibiotics and supportive care. Some form of interventional therapy is required to decompress the biliary tree. This may be by ERCP (usually with sphincterotomy) or by percutaneous transhepatic cholangiography.

PARASITIC DISEASES OF THE HEPATOBILIARY SYSTEM
A variety of tropical parasites may affect the liver and its drainage system. The most common are the flukes *Fasciola hepatica* (**Fig. 9.53**) and *Clonorchis sinensis*.

F. hepatica is widely distributed because its definitive host is the sheep. Human infection usually follows the ingestion of watercress grown in sheep-farming areas. Many infections are asymptomatic. The flukes enter the bile ducts having first traversed the intestinal mucosa and the liver. They may cause intermittent obstruction with symptoms similar to those produced by gallstones. Eosinophilia is common and hepatomegaly occurs. Eggs can be found in the stool or in duodenal aspirates. Praziquantel is the treatment of choice.

Clonorchis (or *Opisthorcis*) *sinensis* is limited to the Far East and is transmitted by eating raw fish. The flukes live in the bile ducts, and symptoms range from none to those of bile duct obstruction (**Fig. 9.54**). Severe, chronic infection may lead to cholangiocarcinoma.

PANCREAS
The pancreas may be involved in systemic diseases such as sepsis, in which pancreatic abscesses occur, although this is rare (**Fig. 9.55**). Most pancreatic infections are secondary to acute pancreatitis caused by gallstones or alcohol. Pancreatic necrosis and associated peritonitis leads to infection with bowel organism. Often, in these cases, surgical debridement is required in addition to antibiotics.

PERITONITIS

Inflammation of the peritoneal cavity is usually due to infection but can be caused by other agents, such as chemicals. Infective causes are usually classed as either primary (i.e. spontaneous) or secondary (to intra-abdominal sepsis).

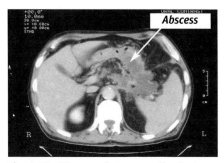

Fig. 9.55 *CT scan of a pancreatic abscess following* Salmonella enteritidis *bacteraemia.*

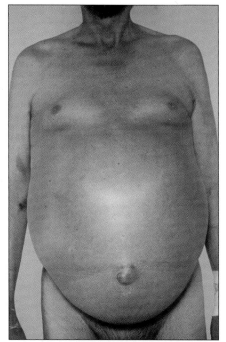

Fig. 9.56 *A patient with gross ascites due to chronic liver disease who is at risk of bacterial peritonitis.*

SPONTANEOUS PERITONITIS

This is most often seen in alcoholic liver disease in association with ascites (**Fig. 9.56**). Other chronic liver diseases and malignant or inflammatory diseases in which ascites is present also increase the risk of peritonitis. Rarely, spontaneous peritonitis may occur in otherwise healthy hosts. Although the pneumococcus and some streptococci may cause peritonitis, most cases in patients with cirrhosis are due to enteric organisms, such as *E. coli* and enterococci. Anaerobes are rarely recovered in these cases.

Patients may have abdominal pain and usually have a fever. There may be vomiting, and signs of peritonitis, such as guarding and rebound tenderness, may be elicited. In patients with chronic liver disease, peritonitis may cause decompensation and encephalopathy. Diagnosis relies on obtaining samples of ascitic fluid for microscopy and culture. Gram stain is often negative. Usually the fluid contains more than 300 leucocytes/mm³ and has a pH <7.35. The fluid may have a raised protein level, but low levels may be seen in liver disease or other hypoalbuminaemic states.

Therapy is usually empiric while cultures are awaited. A third-generation cephalosporin is usually appropriate and treatment can be modified after culture results are available. Failure to improve after 48 hours should prompt a search for another source of sepsis and may necessitate laparotomy.

SECONDARY PERITONITIS

Any focus of intra-abdominal inflammation may lead to peritonitis. The organisms are usually of gastrointestinal origin and include Enterobacteriaceae, anaerobes and enterococci. Occasionally, a genitourinary source may be implicated and organisms such as *Neisseria gonorrhoea* and *Chlamydia* spp. need to be considered.

Patients usually have fever, abdominal pain and vomiting. There may be generalized peritonitis with abdominal rigidity and guarding or there may be localized peritonism, sometimes in association with an abdominal mass, such as an appendix abscess. Gram-negative septic shock may ensue in those who are bacteraemic.

Treatment depends on the underlying cause but parenteral antibiotics are required to cover the suspected organisms. In practice, this usually involves a β-lactamase-stable β-lactam and an aminoglycoside in conjunction with metronidazole to cover anaerobic pathogens.

Peritonitis associated with peritoneal dialysis

Patients receiving continuous ambulatory peritoneal dialysis (CAPD) as renal replacement therapy are at increased risk of peritonitis. The risk arises from having a permanently indwelling Tenckhoff catheter and is increased if aseptic technique in handling the catheter is compromised. Gram-positive cocci (from the skin) are the usual pathogens, with coagulase-negative staphylococci being more common than *S. aureus*. Gram-negative bacilli occur in up to 30% of cases and, occasionally, fungi may be implicated.

Patients with CAPD peritonitis may become unwell with fever and vomiting or they may have only mild abdominal discomfort and notice that the dialysis fluid has become cloudy (**Fig. 9.57**). This reflects the presence of white cells – usually >100 neutrophils/mm^3. The Gram stain is usually negative and the diagnosis rests on culture of the fluid. Bacteraemia is rare.

Treatment can usually be given intraperitoneally via the Tenckhoff catheter. Vancomycin is usually the treatment of choice. Catheter removal is not usually required unless the patient is not responding to the treatment or the infection is due to fungi.

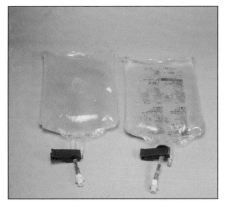

Fig. 9.57 *Cloudy dialysis fluid in chronic ambulatory peritoneal dialysis peritonitis.*

INTRA-ABDOMINAL ABSCESS

Abscesses within the abdominal cavity may occur in a variety of sites and may complicate peritonitis. Conditions leading to abscess formation are shown in **Figure 9.58**. Intra-abdominal sepsis is usually polymicrobial with organisms from bowel. Symptoms may be acute or subacute. Local abdominal symptoms depend on the site and source of the abscess. Pain and fever, often accompanied by rigors, are common, and there may be diarrhoea.

Patients may be bacteraemic but the diagnosis of intra-abdominal abscesses can be difficult and must be considered in the appropriate clinical setting. Newer imaging techniques, such as ultrasound and CT scanning (**Fig. 9.59**), are extremely useful and nowadays preclude the need for exploratory laparotomy. In some centres, radiolabelled leucocyte scans are used to localize abscesses. Although antibiotics are useful to suppress the systemic features of sepsis, surgical (or radiological) drainage of the abscess is the most important procedure (**Fig. 9.60**).

Diseases associated with intra-abdominal abscess

Diverticulitis
Perforated peptic ulcer
Appendicitis
Pancreatitis
Crohn's disease
Trauma

Fig. 9.58 *Diseases associated with intra-abdominal abscess.*

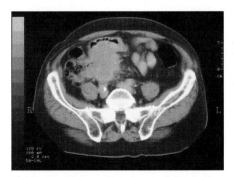

Fig. 9.59 *CT scan of an intra-abdominal abscess secondary to colonic carcinoma.*

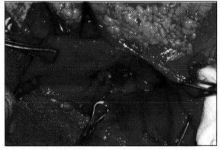

Fig. 9.60 *Pancreatic abscess at laparotomy.*

chapter 10

Urinary and Genital Tract Infections

URINARY TRACT INFECTION

Urinary tract infection (UTI) is a term that encompasses a variety of clinical problems, ranging from asymptomatic bacteriuria through to ascending renal infection and Gram-negative sepsis. Women, at any age, are more at risk of UTI than men and the risk in both sexes increases with age (**Fig. 10.1**). There are a variety of classifications of UTI but a practical one is:
- acute, uncomplicated UTI in women;
- acute, uncomplicated UTI in men;
- complicated UTI in both sexes.

CAUSATIVE ORGANISMS

The vast majority of uncomplicated UTI are caused by *Escherichia coli*. There are only a limited number of *E. coli* serotypes that infect the urinary tract and these are sometimes referred to as uropathogenic strains. Other Gram-negative bacteria, such as *Proteus* spp. and *Klebsiella* spp., occasionally cause UTI. *Staphylococcus saprophyticus* may cause uncomplicated UTI in young women but it rarely causes ascending infection (**Fig. 10.2**) .

E. coli is also the most common pathogen in complicated UTI, but it is much less prevalent in this setting. Other organisms that are frequently involved are other Enterobacteriaceae, enterococci, *Pseudomonas* spp. and coagulase-negative staphylococci (other than *S. saprophyticus*). In catheterized patients, particularly if they have received antibiotics, yeasts are a not uncommon finding.

Prevalence of UTI in different age groups		
	Male	**Females**
Children	<1%	5%
Young adults	<1%	15 - 20%
Middle-aged	10 - 20%	15 - 30%
Elderly	10 - 30%	15 - 40%

Notes:
* Risk increased in adult women because of sexual intercourse and gynaecological surgery
* Middle-aged and older men are at increasing risk of UTI due to prostatic hypertrophy
* The elderly are more likely to be catheterized for urinary incontinence

Fig. 10.1 *Prevalence of urinary tract infection at different ages.*

Organisms commonly associated with urinary tract infections (UTI)

Escherichia coli	esp. uncomplicated UTI
Staphylococcus saprophyticus	esp. cystitis in young adult women
Proteus mirabilis	sometimes associated with renal stones
Klebsiella sp.	
Enterobacter sp.	
Pseudomonas aeruginosa	esp. nosocomial UTI
Staphylococcus epidermidis	
Candida sp.	associated with urinary catheterization

Fig. 10.2 *Common causes of urinary tract infection.*

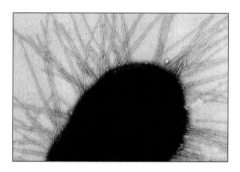

Fig. 10.3 *Fimbriae in* Escherichia coli *shown by electron microscopy.*

PATHOGENESIS

The normal perineum and anterior urethra are usually colonized with a variety of bacteria. Most community-acquired UTI result from these bacteria ascending the urethra to reach the bladder. Haematogenous or lymphatic spread of organisms to the bladder is relatively rare.

E. coli usually colonizes the perineum, vaginal introitus and the urethra before causing infection. There are undoubtedly host differences; for example, it may be that oestrogens promote perineal and urethral colonization in women. Uropathogenic strains may have an advantage over others in terms of their ability to adhere urothelial cells through a variety of adhesions, the best studied of which are the *P fimbriae* (**Fig. 10.3**).

CLINICAL FEATURES

In neonates and young children the clinical features of UTI are nonspecific, and affected children may present with fever and vomiting. Older children and adults usually have localizing signs. The elderly may, like children, present nonspecifically with fever and confusion.

Acute uncomplicated cystitis

This occurs most commonly in young women but it also occurs in older children and in older adults of both sexes. Lower UTI usually presents with the frequent passage of small amounts of turbid urine. Voiding is often painful and there may be accompanying suprapubic or pelvic discomfort. The urine may smell offensive and sometimes it is frankly bloodstained. Systemic symptoms, such as fever, are rare. However, up to 30% of patients presenting with acute lower UTI may have occult upper tract (renal) infection.

Acute pyelonephritis

Ascending infection affects the renal parenchyma. This is more common if lower tract UTI persists untreated for more than 1 week or if there has been a recent UTI. Acute pyelonephritis most commonly presents with fever, rigors and flank pain in association with lower tract symptoms, such as frequency and dysuria. Patients with ascending infection may be only moderately unwell but can present with Gram-negative sepsis.

Complicated urinary tract infection

Whereas acute cystitis and pyelonephritis predominantly occur in young women with anatomically normal urinary tracts, people with structural or functional abnormalities of the urinary tract are said to have complicated UTI (**Fig. 10.4**). Most men and patients of both sexes with indwelling urinary catheters have complicated infections as well.

This group of patients may have nonspecific symptoms and signs that localize poorly to the urinary tract. More importantly, complicated UTI presents particular issues when it comes to management, such as the duration of therapy or the utility of prophylaxis.

DIAGNOSIS

Methods based on culture

The diagnosis of UTI is made by confirming the presence of bacteria in the urine by culture. In infants, urine can be obtained from suprapubic aspiration of the bladder under sterile conditions. In older patients, an 'in-out' bladder catheter can be passed *per urethra*. In practice, most urine specimens are obtained by voiding, which means that there is a risk of contamination of the specimen with perineal bacteria, especially in women. This risk can be minimized by obtaining a mid-stream urine specimen after cleansing the genital area. Quantitative culture and specific identification of the organisms detected help to distinguish urinary pathogens from contaminants (**Fig. 10.5**). Usually contaminants are present in low numbers and are polymicrobial; they are not normally pathogenic bacteria.

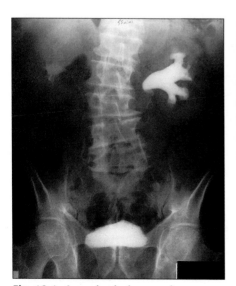

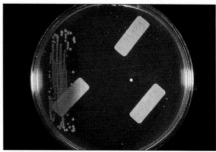

Fig. 10.5 *Colonies of* Escherichia coli *on agar.*

Fig. 10.4 *A renal calculus seen in an intravenous urogram.*

Traditionally, following the work of Kass, the detection of 10^5 bacteria or colony-forming units per millilitre of urine is considered diagnostic of a UTI in asymptomatic patients. However, women with symptomatic acute UTI may have lower counts of recognized urinary pathogens and will respond to appropriate therapy. It is now clear that, in patients with symptoms, the finding of $>10^3$ CFU/ml is significant and sufficient for diagnosing a UTI. Thus, the actual level of bacteriuria should be considered in the light of the clinical setting.

Nonculture methods

More rapid detection of infection allows more rapid treatment and avoids the delay of 24–48 hours before cultures become positive. Microscopic haematuria can occur in up to 60% of UTI and may be a useful pointer in symptomatic patients. However, it is insufficiently sensitive to be used as a diagnostic test. The presence of leucocytes in the urine (pyuria) is highly associated with UTI, and the absence of pyuria makes UTI highly unlikely (**Fig. 10.6**). Pyuria is less common in complicated and catheter-associated UTI. Microscopic detection of leucocytes is variably sensitive, depending on whether the specimen is centrifuged or not. Bacteria seen on microscopy of Gram-stained, unspun urine is a specific but insensitive indicator of UTI.

New dipstick technology provides a rapid test for the presence of bacteria and leucocytes in the urine. The stick detects pyuria by changing colour in the presence of leucocyte esterase, and the presence of nitrites indicates bacterial breakdown (**Fig. 10.7**). In many institutions, urine specimens can be screened by dipstick and only those that are positive for nitrites or leucocytes are submitted for culture and further work-up. However, any patient suspected of having a complicated UTI should have a specimen sent for culture, regardless of the dipstick result.

TREATMENT

Although various nonspecific measures are recommended for treating UTI, probably the only useful one is to maintain a good fluid intake. The fluid may help to dilute bacteria in the urine, with increased urinary flow rates reducing bacterial adhesion. This may provide some symptomatic relief. However, most symptomatic UTI should be treated with antibiotics. The choice of agent depends on the pathogen, but therapy is usually started empirically before cultures are available. The prescriber must be aware of the local resistance patterns among coliforms and other organisms that cause UTI.

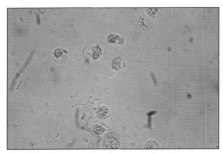

Fig. 10.6 *Pus cells seen in urine microscopy.*

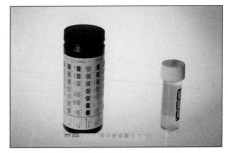

Fig. 10.7 *Urine dipstick positive for nitrites and leucocytes.*

Acute symptomatic cystitis

Acute symptomatic cystitis will usually respond to a short course of oral antibiotics. A 3-day course is probably as good as a 7-day course and both are better than the previously popular single dose therapy for UTI.

Acute pyelonephritis

The therapeutic approach to acute pyelonephritis depends on the severity of the disease. Some patients can be managed on an outpatient basis with oral agents but many will require 48–72 hours of parenteral therapy before oral therapy can be used reliably. Antibiotics are usually continued for at least 14 days.

Complicated urinary tract infection

For complicated UTI, at least 14 days of treatment are needed, sometimes with a prolonged course of parenteral antibiotics, depending on the infecting organism and the severity of the disease. For males who relapse, prolonged antimicrobial therapy (6–8 weeks) may be required.

Asymptomatic bacteriuria

Asymptomatic bacteriuria rarely requires treatment. Exceptions include children, who should be treated and investigated. Also, pregnant women with bacteriuria have an increased risk of pyelonephritis, which may adversely affect the outcome of the pregnancy, so they should also be screened routinely and treated. Neutropenic patients and those who are immunosuppressed, particularly renal transplant recipients, should be treated in order to minimize the risk of ascending or disseminated infection.

Catheter-related infections

Catheter-related infections are common in hospitals, with the risk of bacteriuria increasing with the duration of catheterization (**Fig. 10.8**). Most cases are asymptomatic and do not require treatment. However, symptomatic infections should be treated with systemic antibiotics and, if possible, removal of the catheter. Antibiotics are usually given for 7 days.

PROPHYLAXIS

Some women are prone to recurrent UTI and although some cases may be related to sexual intercourse, the majority are not. Women with two or more episodes per year may adopt various strategies:
- continuous low-dose antimicrobial prophylaxis;
- self-administered single dose prophylaxis at the onset of symptoms; or
- single postcoital dose prophylaxis if UTI are temporally related to sexual intercourse.

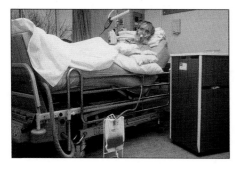

Fig. 10.8 *Patient with a urinary catheter.*

Infections related to indwelling urinary catheters can be reduced by using closed collecting systems and paying meticulous attention to aseptic technique when handling catheter, tubing and bag. Antibiotic prophylaxis tends to lead to colonization with resistant strains.

ABSCESSES

RENAL ABSCESS

Sometimes referred to as renal carbuncles, abscesses that arise in the renal cortex usually result from blood-borne spread of bacteria to the kidney. The vast majority are due to *Staphylococcus aureus* and are usually single, unilateral abscesses.

Renal cortical abscesses usually present with flank pain and fever, sometimes with rigors. They are more common in men. Communication with the renal collecting system is rare and urinalysis is therefore usually negative. Clinical examination is usually unrewarding but occasionally there is a bulge in the flank overlying the abscess.

Renal medullary abscesses usually arise from infected urine in the presence of some urinary tract abnormality. The common problems associated with medullary abscesses are vesicoureteric reflux and obstruction, the latter most commonly seen with renal calculi. In addition, people with diabetes mellitus are more prone to medullary abscesses. Unlike cortical abscesses, those involving the medulla (**Fig. 10.9**) are usually caused by urinary pathogens, such as *E. coli*, *Klebsiella* spp. or *Proteus* spp.

XANTHOGRANULOMATOUS PYELONEPHRITIS

Rarely, chronic UTI or obstructive uropathy may be associated with severe intrarenal inflammation and abscess formation in a condition called xanthogranulomatous pyelonephritis. The abscess cavity solidifies and is made up of a yellow, lipid-laden substance. Histologically, there are chronic inflammatory cells and macrophages stuffed with cholesterol and other lipids (**Fig. 10.10**).

Clinically, fever and flank pain are the most common features. In contrast to cortical abscesses due to *S. aureus*, many of these patients also have some urinary symptoms and have abnormalities on urinalysis. In cases of xanthogranulomatous pyelonephritis, there may be chronic systemic upset with malaise and weight loss.

PERINEPHRIC ABSCESS

Most of these abscesses arise from the rupture of an intrarenal abscess into the perinephric fat. Thus, the causative organisms are usually *S. aureus* (from cortical abscesses) or Gram-negative bacilli (from corticomedullary abscesses). Sometimes anaerobes or fungi may be involved.

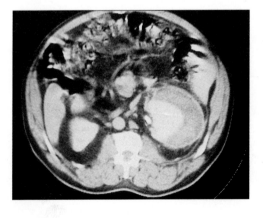

Fig. 10.9 *CT scan showing corticomedullary abscess due to* **Escherichia coli.**

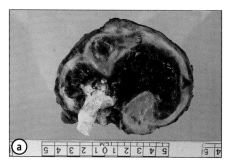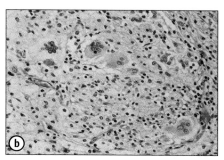

Fig. 10.10 *Xanthogranulomatous pyelonephritis: (a) nephrectomy specimen; (b) histological appearance.*

A perinephric abscess may be difficult to diagnose because the presentation is often insidious. There may be fever and loin pain, but both may occur late. As the abscess expands, the diaphragm may become involved, leading to pleuritic pain and sometimes a pleural effusion. The psoas muscle may also become inflamed, with pain referred to the hip. Blood and urine cultures can be positive but not invariably.

DIAGNOSIS

The diagnosis of abscesses associated with the kidney depends on some form of imaging. Ultrasound and computed tomography (CT) scanning are now the most commonly used methods. These methods can usually distinguish an abscess from a simple cyst or from a renal tumour. Blood tests are nonspecific and urinalysis may be unhelpful.

MANAGEMENT

Treatment relies on adequate antimicrobial therapy, usually in conjunction with some form of drainage procedure. Open surgical drainage is less common now that percutaneous ultrasound or CT-guided drainage is widely available (**Fig. 10.11**). Antibiotics need to be given for at least 4 weeks, administered parenterally for the first 2 weeks. The kidney is usually irreversibly damaged in xanthogranulomatous pyelonephritis and most cases require nephrectomy.

RENAL TUBERCULOSIS

Tuberculosis can affect any part of the genitourinary tract and many patients with pulmonary tuberculosis may have asymptomatic renal involvement. About half of those

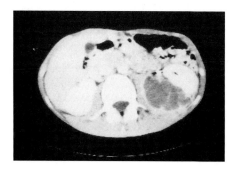

Fig. 10.11 *Left perinephric abscess on a CT scan.*

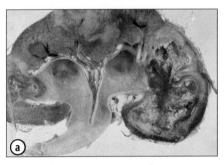

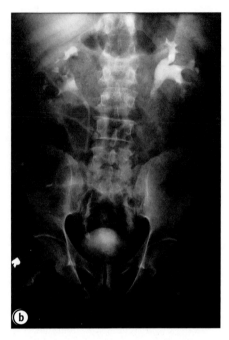

Fig. 10.12 *Renal tract tuberculosis:*
(a) gross specimen; (b) beading of ureters
seen in an intravenous urogram.

presenting with renal tuberculosis have evidence of disease elsewhere, usually in the lungs. Renal tuberculosis is more common in the elderly. Most patients have few symptoms so diagnosis can be difficult. Some patients have symptoms related to the renal tract and some have loin pain. Constitutional upset is rare.

Analysis of the urine frequently shows microscopic, and occasionally frank, haematuria and pyuria. Ultrasound scanning and intravenous urography are usually abnormal, with most cases manifesting unilateral disease. Renal function is rarely impaired. Diagnosis may be made from culture of early morning urine specimens, biopsy material or by finding acid-fast bacilli elsewhere in the presence of typical urinary tract abnormalities (**Fig. 10.12**).

Treatment is with standard antituberculous therapy for at least 9 months. Occasionally, surgery is required for complications, such as ureteric scarring.

PROSTATIC INFECTIONS

ACUTE BACTERIAL PROSTATITIS

The prostate gland may become infected by several routes:

- ascending urethral infection;
- reflux of infected urine into prostatic ducts;
- lymphatic or direct spread from the rectum; or
- haematogenous spread.

Causative organisms

The types of organisms involved are similar to those that cause UTI, with *E. coli* predominating. Other Enterobacteriaceae and *Pseudomonas* spp. are not infrequently the cause. *S. aureus* may lead to prostatic infection following bacteraemia but other Gram-positive organisms rarely cause acute prostatitis. Prostatitis may be a consequence of urinary catheters in hospital.

Clinical features

The clinical features of acute bacterial prostatitis are typically an acute onset of fever and rigors in association with back or suprapubic pain. Affected men may have urinary frequency or may have symptoms suggestive of outflow obstruction. Rectal examination reveals a warm, tender prostate, which may be swollen. Urinalysis is usually abnormal and bacteriuria is a frequent finding. An acutely swollen prostate may also be demonstrated by ultrasound imaging (**Fig. 10.13**).

Management

Treatment is with antibiotics that penetrate prostatic tissue well, such as trimethoprim or the fluoroquinolones. β-lactam antibiotics do not normally get into prostatic secretions in very high concentrations but are probably able to in acute infection. Treatment should continue for at least 4–6 weeks to ensure cure and reduce the risk of chronic prostatitis.

CHRONIC BACTERIAL PROSTATITIS

Unlike acute infections, chronic bacterial prostatitis can be difficult to diagnose because it is more variable in presentation. A similar range of organisms is involved, however. Some patients may present without symptoms when bacteriuria is discovered incidentally. Others may have preceding bouts of acute prostatitis. Most patients, however, have some symptoms of UTI or prostatic irritation, such as urgency and frequency. They may also have low-grade perineal or low back pain. Patients may present with recurrent or relapsing UTI. Clinical examination is unhelpful and, in particular, prostatic examination is usually normal.

Most men have prostatic calculi and these may be the nidus of infection in chronic bacterial prostatitis (**Fig. 10.14**). Although symptoms of UTI may settle with antibiotics as the urine becomes sterile, antibiotics tend not to penetrate the prostate well and bacteria infecting the calculi in the prostate are not affected. These organisms can then cause relapses of the symptoms.

Making a bacteriological diagnosis in chronic bacterial prostatitis can be difficult but is helped by using the bacterial localization cultures introduced by Stamey and others. The first 10ml of voided urine is collected (VB1) as is a mid-stream urine sample (VB2) and both are sent for culture. The patient's prostate gland is then massaged *per rectum* and the few drops of expressed prostatic secretions (EPS) are collected and cultured, as are the first 10ml of voided urine after prostatic massage (VB3) (**Fig. 10.15**). Cultures are done

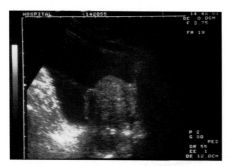

Fig. 10.13 *Swollen prostate in acute prostatitis seen on ultrasound.*

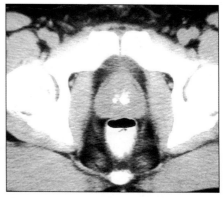

Fig. 10.14 *CT scan showing prostatic calculi.*

Fig. 10.15 *The Stamey test for prostatitis.*

Principles of diagnosis of prostatitis

VB$_1$ - first 5-10 ml urine voided (represents urethral flow)

VB$_2$ - mid-stream urine sample (represents bladder urine)

Prostatic massage

Expressed prostatic secretion

Microscope slide

VB$_3$ - Urine sample voided after prostatic massage

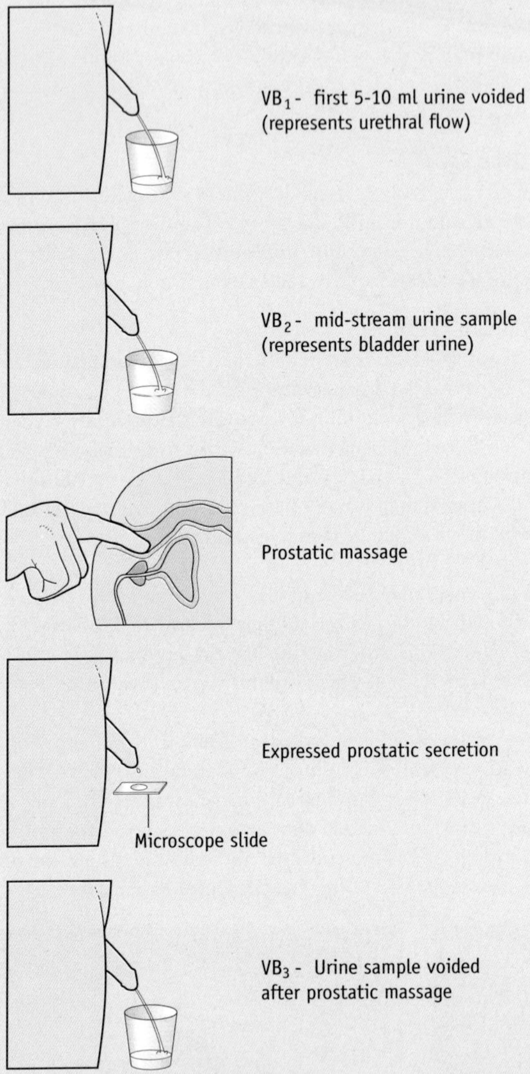

① If EPS or VB$_3$ show >10 white cells per high power field, bacterial prostatitis is likely; this is strengthened by the finding of lipid-laden macrophages

② If the colony count of bacteria cultured from the EPS or VB$_3$ is greater than 10x the colony count from VB$_1$, prostatitis is likely

N.B. VB$_1$ should be free of white cells; i.e. urethritis must be absent for a diagnosis of prostatitis to be made

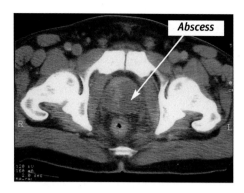

Abscess

Fig. 10.16 *CT scan of a prostatic abscess.*

quantitatively so that the concentration of bacteria in the various samples can be compared. Bacterial counts in chronic bacterial prostatitis are highest in the EPS and VB3 specimens, but if there is urethral infection or colonization, counts in the VB1 specimen will be high.

Treatment of chronic prostatitis requires antibiotics with good access to prostatic secretions. Agents such as trimethoprim or ciprofloxacin should be given for at least 4 weeks and sometimes for as long as 3 months. Patients with large prostatic stones may require surgery. In some cases of chronic prostatitis, cure may not be possible but low-dose, long-term suppressive antibiotics may help control symptoms.

PROSTATIC ABSCESS

Occasionally, acute bacterial prostatitis may not resolve completely and may go on to abscess formation (**Fig. 10.16**). Abscesses may also arise from blood-borne infections, as may occur with *S. aureus*. In patients infected with the human immunodeficiency virus (HIV), abscesses caused by *Cryptococcus neoformans* have been described. Prostatic abscesses may present with localizing symptoms or with a fever of unknown origin. Surgical drainage is usually required.

EPIDIDYMITIS

Infections of the epididymis arise in two ways:
* as a sexually transmitted disease in association with urethritis in young men; and
* in association with UTI or prostatitis in older men.

Sexually transmitted epididymitis is most commonly due to *Chlamydia trachomatis* or to *Neisseria gonorrhoeae*. The second type of epididymitis is usually caused by coliforms or *Pseudomonas* spp.

Whatever the cause, the clinical presentation is of painful, unilateral swelling of the scrotum (**Fig. 10.17**). Often the testis is involved so it is not possible to distinguish the epididymis from the testis when palpating the inflammatory scrotal mass. There may be associated urethral discharge and abnormalities on urinalysis.

Urethral swabs should be sent for microscopy and gonococcal culture, and urine should be cultured. Treatment depends on the cause but should include cover for *Chlamydia* and gonorrhoea in sexually active young men.

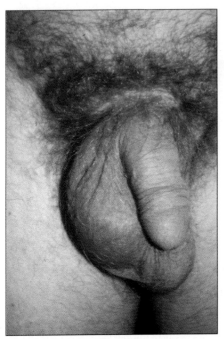

Fig. 10.17 *Right epididymo-orchitis.*

Causes of epididymo-orchitis

Neisseria gonorrhoeae
Chlamydia trachomatis
Escherichia coli
Pseudomonas aeruginosa
Mycobacterium tuberculosis
Brucella melitensis
Mumps virus
Coxsackie B virus
Blastomyces dermatitidis

Fig. 10.18 *Causes of epididymo-orchitis.*

ORCHITIS

The testis may become involved in epididymitis, as described above, but it is more commonly infected by blood-borne pathogens. Mumps is the most common cause of orchitis but others are listed in **Figure 10.18**. Patients present with unilateral pain and swelling. Differentiation from torsion of the testis or from tumours is aided by testicular ultrasound. The testis affected by viral orchitis may atrophy.

SEXUALLY TRANSMITTED DISEASES

The classical sexually transmitted diseases (STDs) are syphilis, gonorrhoea and chancroid, but a wide variety of pathogens are sexually transmissible (**Fig. 10.19**). Any person who is sexually active is at risk of acquiring an STD but numerous studies have shown that the risk is highest in urban areas, in low socioeconomic groups, in the young and in association with illicit drug use and prostitution.

Patients with symptomatic STD usually seek treatment early but a variety of infections are relatively asymptomatic, especially in women, favouring spread of infection. The principles of STD management rely on:

- accurate and rapid diagnosis;
- adequate treatment;
- confirmation of cure; and
- follow-up and treatment of contacts.

Sexually transmissible infections

Syphilis Gonorrhoea Chancroid	legally defined sexually transmitted diseases in the UK
Bacterial infections	
Chlamydia trachomatis	non-gonococcal urethritis pelvic inflammatory disease lymphogranuloma venereum
Ureaplasma urealyticum	non-gonococcal urethritis
Haemophilus ducreyi	granuloma inguinale
Viral infections	
Herpes simplex (types 1 and 2) Papilloma virus Molluscum contagiosum HIV Hepatitis A* Hepatitis B Hepatitis C	genital warts
Protozoan infections	
Trichomonas vaginalis Giardia lamblia* Entamoeba histolytica*	
Others	
Candida species Pubic lice Scabies	

*These infections are faecal-orally transmitted and are more common in homosexual men

Fig. 10.19 *Sexually transmissible infections.*

Patients presenting with a suspected STD should be screened for other infections because multiple infections are not uncommon. Management should involve some form of counselling about STD risks, particularly in this HIV era.

The presentation of STDs can be very variable but patients generally present with genital discharge, genital ulcers, genital swelling or pelvic or perineal discomfort.

GONORRHOEA

Gonorrhoea is caused by *Neisseria gonorrhoeae*. It usually presents with genital discharge and dysuria. However, infection can be asymptomatic, particularly in women. Rectal and pharyngeal infections are not uncommon in women and homosexual men and are frequently asymptomatic.

Local infection

Urethritis in men is the most common presentation, with symptoms arising within 2–5 days of infection (**Fig. 10.20**). There is a purulent discharge and dysuria. Complications, such as epididymitis and periurethral abscess, can occur.

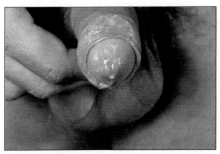

Fig. 10.20 *Gonococcal urethritis in a male.*

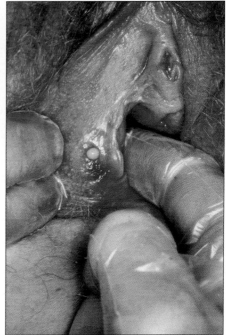

Fig. 10.21 *Gonococcal infection of Bartholin's gland.*

Women usually have a primary infection of the uterine cervix which is, most of the time, asymptomatic (**Fig. 10.21**). Some women may complain of vaginal discharge and some may develop urethritis and symptoms suggestive of UTI. Local complications include the development of a Bartholin's abscess, but the most important complication is pelvic inflammatory disease (PID).

Anorectal disease

Up to half of women with genital gonorrhoea have positive rectal cultures for *N. gonorrhoeae*, probably as a result of local contamination by vaginal secretions. Rectal gonorrhoea may result from anal intercourse in women or homosexual men. Most infections are asymptomatic but some patients may have an acute proctitis with discharge and rectal bleeding.

Other sites of infection

Oral sex may lead to carriage of *N. gonorrhoeae* in the throat with the potential for transmission to the genitals. Pharyngeal infection is usually asymptomatic.

Eye infections in the neonate may arise if the mother has active gonorrhoea at the time of delivery. This usually presents as a mucopurulent conjunctivitis and must be differentiated from that due to *S. aureus* or *C. trachomatis*.

Gonorrhoea is a cause of pelvic inflammatory disease through ascending infection. Rarely, acute perihepatitis (Fitz-Hugh–Curtis syndrome) occurs when infection spreads via the fallopian tube to the liver capsule and adjacent peritoneum. Affected patients have pain in the right upper quadrant and fever as well as signs of PID. Laparoscopy may reveal adhesions between the liver and the peritoneum (**Fig. 10.22**).

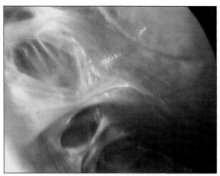

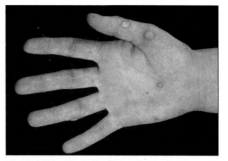

Fig. 10.22 *Perihepatitis with gonorrhoea.*

Fig. 10.23 *Rash in disseminated gonococcal infection.*

Disseminated gonococcal infection

In about 1% of cases, the gonococcus becomes invasive and a bacteraemia develops, leading to disseminated gonococcal infection. The most common manifestations are skin rash and an asymmetrical polyarthritis (**Fig. 10.23**). The rash usually involves the distal extremities, particularly the hands, and is most commonly in the form of a few pustules on a red base. The arthritis most commonly affects the knees, hands and wrists. Polymorphs are present in the synovial fluid and about one-quarter of cases are culture positive from the joint. Gonococcal endocarditis is an extremely rare complication of disseminated gonococcal infection.

Diagnosis of gonorrhoea

Diagnosis traditionally rests on the demonstration of Gram-negative diplococci within polymorphs on microscopy and confirmation by culture. Gram staining is a rapid and, in symptomatic cases of urethritis, sensitive method of diagnosis (**Fig. 10.24**). Sensitivity is lower in asymptomatic disease and in rectal and pharyngeal infections. Culture remains the gold standard. *N. gonorrhoeae* is a delicate organism so care must be taken when obtaining specimens for culture. Ideally, specimens should be plated out immediately. Increasingly, molecular methods of diagnosis such as polymerase chain reaction are being used.

Principles of treatment

Most strains of *N. gonorrhoeae* are sensitive to penicillin but over the past 20 years strains resistant to penicillin have emerged, particularly in the Far East and Africa. Most of the resistant strains produce a plasmid-mediated β-lactamase and are termed penicillinase-producing *N. gonorrhoeae* (PPNG). Chromosomal resistance, not due to β-lactamase, also occurs.

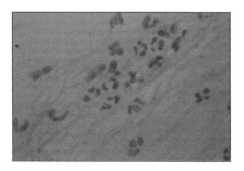

Fig. 10.24 *Microscopy of urethral discharge in gonorrhoea.*

139

Unless local rates of PPNG are high, most cases of uncomplicated gonorrhoea can be treated with a single oral dose of an antibiotic such as azithromycin or high-dose amoxycillin or with a single parenteral dose of ceftriaxone. Quinolones or spectinomycin can be used for PPNG, depending on sensitivities. Many clinics routinely screen and test for cure 1 week after treatment.

Patients with disseminated gonococcal infection or PID may occasionally require hospitalization initially and treatment with parenteral antibiotics. Polymicrobial infection is common in PID and therefore anaerobes and chlamydiae should be treated as well.

Whenever possible, sexual contacts of patients with gonorrhoea should be screened. Many centres advocate 'epidemiological' treatment of these contacts as the risk of gonorrhoea is high and they may not return to the clinic for follow-up.

NONGONOCOCCAL URETHRITIS AND *CHLAMYDIA TRACHOMATIS*

Most cases of nongonococcal urethritis (NGU) are due to infection with *C. trachomatis*, an obligate intracellular bacterium. Infection with *C. trachomatis* is now one of the most common STDs, probably because many infections are asymptomatic. Other causes of NGU include *Mycoplasma hominis* and *Ureaplasma urealyticum*.

Clinical features

Nongonococcal urethritis is less severe than gonococcal urethritis, with a less purulent discharge. Most women with NGU or with cervicitis due to *C. trachomatis* are asymptomatic. Urethritis is a frequent sequel to treated gonorrhoea and most cases of postgonococcal urethritis are due to *Chlamydia*. Rectal infections occur in homosexual men but are usually asymptomatic.

Complications of chlamydial infection include epididymitis and endometritis, but salpingitis is regarded as the most important. About 25% of cases of acute salpingitis are due to *C. trachomatis* and this infection has been implicated in tubal damage and infertility following asymptomatic salpingitis.

Diagnosis

Diagnosis of chlamydial infection and other causes of NGU is difficult. In the clinic, NGU is frequently diagnosed by semiquantitative assessments of polymorphs in urine or urethral swabs (**Fig. 10.25**); the threshold number of polymorphs depends on the method used. Culture of *C. trachomatis* is now possible but is not always available. Nonculture antigen detection systems are more commonly used and these include immunofluorescence and enzyme-linked immunosorbent assays (**Fig. 10.26**). Increasingly, molecular methods of diagnosis are used. Testing urine specimens for chlamydiae using the ligase chain reaction is starting to become the 'gold standard' in some countries.

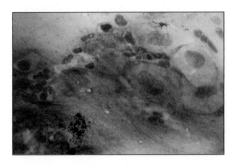

Fig. 10.25 *Pus cells on microscopy of urethral discharge in nongonococcal urethritis.*

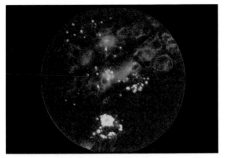

Fig. 10.26 *Positive immunofluorescent test in chlamydial urethritis.*

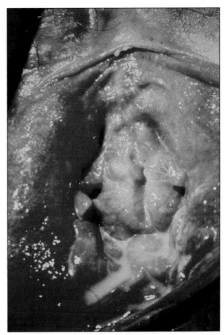

Fig. 10.27 *Vaginal candidiasis.*

Treatment

Chlamydiae and the other causes of NGU are sensitive to tetracyclines and macrolides. Common drugs used are tetracycline, doxycycline, erythromycin and azithromycin. Azithromycin can be given as a single dose but with the other agents treatment is usually needed for at least 1 week.

VAGINITIS

Vulvovaginal candidiasis

Yeasts are common commensals of the vagina but may proliferate and cause symptoms. Yeast infections are more common in the presence of antibiotic therapy, diabetes mellitus, pregnancy, oral contraceptives and glucocorticoid therapy. Most infections are caused by *Candida albicans* but other *Candida* spp. can also cause vaginitis.

Symptoms of candidiasis include itching, sometimes dysuria, vaginal discharge and superficial dyspareunia. Examination reveals inflammation of the vulva and vagina, and a whitish discharge is often present (**Fig. 10.27**). Sometimes plaques of *Candida* appear on the vaginal epithelium.

Diagnosis is made by finding yeasts on wet mount preparations or on Gram stain; this is confirmed by culture of *C. albicans* or other *Candida* spp. Treatment is usually with topical antifungal agents such as nystatin or clotrimazole. Newer systemic imidazoles are also effective but more expensive.

Trichomoniasis

Vaginitis may be due to the protozoan parasite, *Trichomonas vaginalis*. Up to one-half of infected women are asymptomatic. The most common symptom is vaginal discharge, often with some local pruritus. The flagellated organism is visible, along with increased numbers

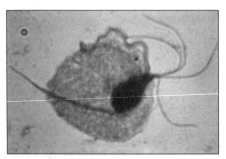

Fig. 10.28 **Trichomonas vaginalis** *seen on a wet mount.*

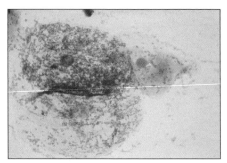

Fig. 10.29 *Clue cells on microscopy of vaginal discharge.*

of polymorphs, on wet mount preparations of vaginal discharge and may be found in the urine (**Fig. 10.28**). Culture on special medium is possible. Treatment is with metronidazole or tinidazole; some strains are now resistant to metronidazoles. Treatment of male partners at the same time is important because most cases are sexually acquired.

Bacterial vaginosis

Sometimes referred to as nonspecific vaginitis, bacterial vaginosis is caused by anaerobic bacteria, most commonly by *Gardnerella vaginalis*. Other anaerobes probably act synergistically to produce inflammation. Although many infections are asymptomatic, patients usually complain of a vaginal discharge with a 'fishy' odour. The odour is due to the volatile amines produced by the metabolism of *G. vaginalis* as the vaginal pH rises.

The diagnosis is made by demonstrating the vaginal pH to be greater than 4.5, the presence of a thin vaginal discharge, and the presence of clue cells on microscopy (**Fig. 10.29**). Clue cells are epithelial cells with numerous adherent bacteria. Treatment is with metronidazole or clindamycin. Recently, topical clindamycin has been used.

Bacterial vaginosis has been associated with premature rupture of the membranes and an increased risk of post-Caesarean endometritis.

Male partners in cases of vaginitis

Apart from trichomoniasis, there is little evidence to show that either candidal or bacterial vaginosis are primarily sexually transmitted. However, in relapsed or recurrent cases, it is prudent to treat the male partner at the same time as treating the index case.

SYPHILIS

Infection with *Treponema pallidum* can lead to a variety of clinical sequelae. After initial inoculation, this spirochaete reproduces locally and, at the same time, disseminates via the lymphatic vessels.

Primary syphilis

A lesion appears at the inoculation site 2–3 weeks after inoculation. It usually starts as a small papule and then ulcerates to form a painless ulcer, or chancre (**Fig. 10.30**). Chancres usually occur on the genitals but they may occur on the perineum, in the anus or on the mouth. Rectal or cervical chancres usually go unnoticed. Whatever the site, there is often local lymphadenopathy. Untreated, the chancre heals within 1–2 months.

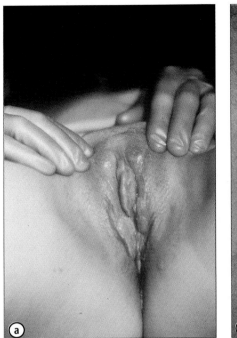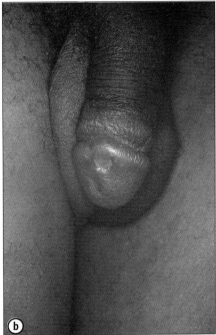

Fig. 10.30 *Primary syphilis: (a) chancre in a female; (b) chancre in a male.*

Secondary syphilis

The clinical features of secondary syphilis follow the dissemination of the spirochaete, usually 4–10 weeks after the first appearance of the chancre. Almost any organ system can be affected, although a rash and lymphadenopathy are very common (**Fig. 10.31**). The clinical features are outlined in **Figure 10.32**. Patients at this stage of disease are highly infectious.

Latent syphilis

If untreated, secondary syphilis resolves over a period of several weeks and is followed by an asymptomatic latent stage. The latent stage is sometimes divided into early latent disease if it occurs within 1 year of the secondary stage and late latent disease if there have been no symptoms or signs of relapse for more than 1 year.

Tertiary syphilis

Late syphilitic symptoms and signs sometimes appear 2 years or more after the initial infection. It is categorized as:

- benign late syphilis;
- cardiac syphilis; or
- neurological syphilis.

All forms of late syphilis are very rare in the antibiotic era, presumably because incidental exposure to antibiotics modifies the course of the disease.

Benign late syphilis is characterized by the presence of gummas; granulomatous lesions of the skin or soft tissues. Sometimes a gumma forms in bone or the viscera, causing local pain or swelling.

143

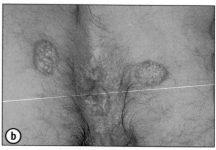

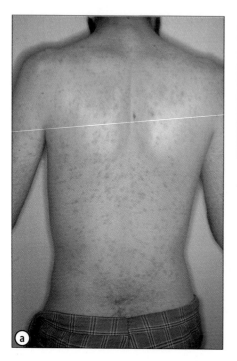

Fig. 10.31 *Secondary syphilis: (a) typical rash; (b) condylomata lata.*

Cardiac syphilis most commonly results in an inflammatory aortitis, sometimes leading to an aneurysm of the ascending aorta (**Fig. 10.33**). The coronary ostia may be involved, leading to ischaemic heart disease.

Neurosyphilis can cause tabes dorsalis or may lead to a dementia. Various degrees of psychosis may occur.

Diagnosis

Various stages of syphilis may be diagnosed clinically but confirmation of the diagnosis by laboratory tests is essential. In primary syphilis, the best way of diagnosing the disease is by finding characteristic treponemes in the fluid from the chancre. This is done using dark ground microscopy and is highly sensitive and specific.

Other stages of syphilis rely on serological tests for diagnosis (**Fig. 10.34**). Nonspecific tests include the Venereal Disease Research Laboratory (VDRL), rapid plasma reagin (RPR) and the Wassermann reaction (WR), all of which detect anticardiolipin antibodies. These tests are positive in about 80% of cases of primary syphilis and all cases of secondary syphilis. Although they may be positive in latent and tertiary disease, the titre wanes with time. The titre should also decline following successful treatment of active disease at any stage. False-positive tests occur in a variety of conditions.

The more specific serological tests are the fluorescent treponemal antibody absorption test (FTA-Abs) and the *T. pallidum* haemagglutination test (TPHA). These use *T. pallidum* raised in rabbits as the antigen to detect antibodies in the patient's serum. The FTA-Abs is the first test to become positive in primary syphilis and both this test and the TPHA are positive in high titre in secondary syphilis. The titres may remain high for a long time. Both these tests are usually positive in late disease; if both are negative, late and latent syphilis can essentially be ruled out.

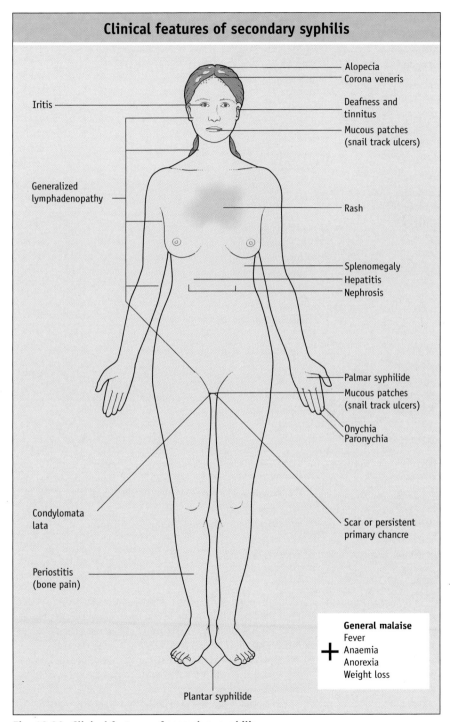

Clinical features of secondary syphilis

Alopecia
Corona veneris

Iritis

Deafness and tinnitus

Mucous patches (snail track ulcers)

Generalized lymphadenopathy

Rash

Splenomegaly
Hepatitis
Nephrosis

Palmar syphilide
Mucous patches (snail track ulcers)

Onychia
Paronychia

Condylomata lata

Scar or persistent primary chancre

Periostitis (bone pain)

General malaise
Fever
Anaemia
Anorexia
Weight loss

Plantar syphilide

Fig. 10.32 *Clinical features of secondary syphilis.*

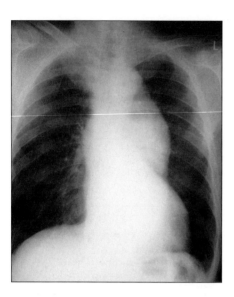

Fig. 10.33 *Thoracic aortic aneurysm in tertiary syphilis.*

Syphilis serology: Interpretation

VDRL or WR	TPHA	FTA-Abs	Interpretation
POS	POS	POS	Untreated or recently treated syphilis or yaws
POS	POS	NEG	A 'problem serum'; needs to be repeated
POS	NEG	POS	A 'problem serum' or primary syphilis
POS	NEG	NEG	False positive*
NEG	NEG	NEG	Uninfected (or incubating very recent infection)
NEG	NEG	POS	Early primary syphilis or old (treated) yaws or syphilis
NEG	POS	NEG	Treated syphilis or false positive TPHA
NEG	POS	POS	Treated early syphilis or untreated or late (treated) syphilis or yaws

*Causes of false-positive VDRL or WR:
  chronic infections; autoimmune disease; malignancy; cirrhosis; old age

Fig. 10.34 *Interpretation of syphilis serology.*

Neurosyphilis presents problems in terms of diagnosis. Although the cerebrospinal fluid (CSF) may have lymphocytes or a raised protein content, it can be normal. The VDRL may be negative in up to a quarter of cases. A positive FTA-Abs or TPHA in the CSF may represent leakage from serum rather than indicating active nervous system infection. Intrathecal production of immunoglobulin (Ig) M antibodies implies active neurological disease and can be detected using a modified test: FTA-Abs IgM. Negative tests for TPHA and FTA-Abs in the CSF excludes neurosyphilis.

There are problems with the serological diagnosis of syphilis in patients who are co-infected with HIV. This is because new infections in these patients may not result in antibody formation and reactivation may be equally difficult to detect.

Treatment

Penicillin has been in use for over 50 years and remains the treatment of choice for syphilis. It still appears to be effective, although the inability to culture *T. pallidum in vitro* precludes antibiotic sensitivity testing. For primary, secondary and early latent syphilis, a single injection or two or three injections, each a week apart, of a long-acting preparation, such as benzathine penicillin, provides adequate treatment. Late latent and tertiary syphilis should be treated with daily injections of aqueous procaine penicillin G for 10 days plus benzathine penicillin G weekly for 3 weeks.

Alternatives to penicillin, for penicillin-allergic patients, include third-generation cephalosporins (e.g. ceftriaxone) and tetracyclines (e.g. doxycycline). Whatever treatment is chosen, adequate doses for a sufficient duration should be enough to comply with national guidelines.

HERPES SIMPLEX VIRUS INFECTIONS

Genital herpes is one of the most common ulcerating diseases of the genitalia. Most cases are caused by herpes simplex virus (HSV) type 2, but some are caused by HSV type 1, the common cause of oral herpes infections. The average incubation time from infection to symptoms is 3–7 days, but over 50% of primary infections are asymptomatic. Primary infection results in latent infection of the sacral root ganglia with the risk of subsequent reactivation, which may cause clinical disease or may be silent.

Clinical features

An attack of genital herpes may have a prodrome of mild constitutional upset with malaise, myalgia and mild fever. This is followed by the appearance of vesicles, which soon break down to leave shallow, painful ulcers (**Figs 10.35** and **10.36**). The external genitalia are

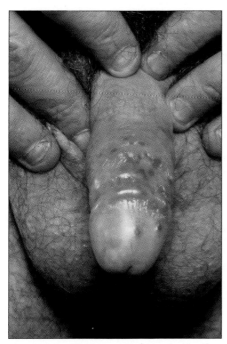

Fig. 10.35 *Primary genital herpes simplex infection in a male.*

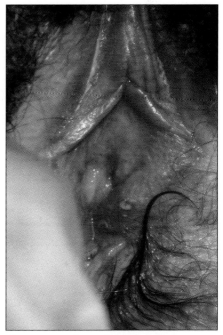

Fig. 10.36 *Primary herpes simplex infection in a female.*

most frequently involved but lesions may be confined to the cervix or to the rectum. There may be associated inguinal lymphadenopathy. The ulcers heal in 2–3 weeks, although healing may be very slow in immunocompromised patients. Primary attacks are usually more severe than recurrent bouts.

Complications are relatively rare, the most common being secondary bacterial or candidal infections. Women may occasionally develop urinary retention. A few patients may develop a mild viral meningitis, usually only with primary attacks. Neonatal HSV infection may occur if the mother is shedding HSV at the time of delivery.

Diagnosis

Diagnosis is usually straightforward. The appearance of typical vesicles and ulcers allows a clinical diagnosis which can be confirmed by culture of HSV type 2 or HSV type 1. In some centres, electron microscopy may be available to make the diagnosis. Serological tests can distinguish HSV type 2 from HSV type 1.

Treatment

Treatment is with systemic antiviral agents such as aciclovir and famciclovir. Such treatment leads to earlier resolution of lesions and symptoms but does not affect the latency of the virus or the risk of recurrences.

GENITAL WARTS

Anogenital warts, or condylomata acuminata, are increasingly common. The causative agent is a deoxyribonucleic acid virus, the human papillomavirus (HPV), which is sexually transmitted. Human papillomavirus types 6, 11, 42, 43 and 44 are associated with genital warts and, sometimes, mild cervical dysplasia. Other types (HPV 16, 18, 31, 33, 35, 39, 45, 51, 52 and 56) are associated with more severe cervical dysplasia and invasive carcinoma of the cervix.

Clinical features

Many infections are asymptomatic but the usual clinical presentation is papules in the anogenital region. Flat warts (aceto-whitening) may be subclinical, whereas papillary, or exophytic, lesions are more obvious to the patient. In females these occur most commonly at the posterior introitus but any part of the perineum may be involved. Lesions may also be confined to the cervix. The penile prepuce is the most common site for warts in uncircumcised men (**Fig. 10.37**). Condylomata acuminata must be distinguished from skin tags, molluscum contagiosum and condylomata lata.

Diagnosis

Human papillomavirus cannot be cultured so diagnosis rests on the clinical appearance of the warts. However, there are now molecular methods of HPV detection. The flat warts stain aceto-white upon application of acetic acid. Biopsy reveals the typical appearance of koilocytosis, or cytoplasmic vacuolization. Koilocytosis may also be seen in cervical smears (**Fig. 10.38**).

Treatment

There is no specific antiviral agent with which to treat HPV infections. Topical chemicals, such as podophylotoxin and trichloroacetic acid, are relatively ineffective, particularly on keratinized skin. Cryotherapy with liquid nitrogen is more effective, and cervical lesions may be treated by laser. Recently, topical interferon therapy has been shown to be effective, but it is expensive. Surgical excision may be required for extensive warts.

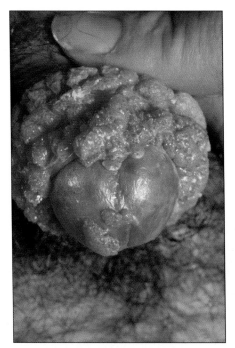

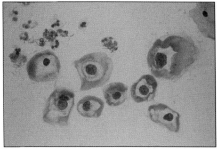

Fig. 10.38 *Cervical smear showing wart inclusions.*

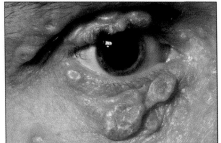

Fig. 10.37 *Genital warts in a male.*

Fig. 10.39 *Characteristic appearance of molluscum contagiosum.*

MOLLUSCUM CONTAGIOSUM

This is a harmless skin condition caused by the largest known human poxvirus and spread by close human contact. Any part of the skin may be involved but genital lesions are usually acquired sexually. The lesions are small, umbilicated papules that usually appear on the genitalia or thighs in sexually acquired disease but may be seen elsewhere on the body (**Fig. 10.39**).

Diagnosis is usually clinical, but viral inclusions may be seen in material expressed from the papules; alternatively, the virus can be identified by electron microscopy.

The papules are usually self-limiting but treatment can accelerate clearance. Common treatments are the local application of phenol into the papule or the use of liquid nitrogen.

ECTOPARASITES

Pediculosis

Pediculosis, or infestation with pubic lice, usually presents with pruritus in the genital and inguinal regions, but other hairy parts of the body can become involved. The causative agent is the human louse *Phthirus pubis* (**Fig. 10.40**). The lice or their eggs (nits) can be found by careful examination of the involved skin and hair. Treatment involves the use of topical malathion or γ-benzene hexachloride with appropriate attention to hygiene. Topical applications should be repeated 1 week after the initial treatment.

Scabies

Scabies is caused by *Sarcoptes scabiei* (**Fig. 10.41**), a mite that is transmitted by close physical contact. The main symptom is pruritus, which is often worse at night. The mite

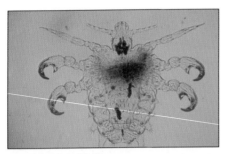

Fig. 10.40 *Pubic louse.*

Fig. 10.41 **Sarcoptes scabiei.**

Fig. 10.42 *Crusted (Norwegian) scabies in a patient with HIV infection.*

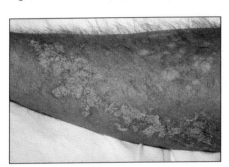

burrows into the skin and causes papules, usually around the wrists and interdigital clefts. Excoriation is a common feature. Any part of the body may be involved except the head and neck. A variant, called Norwegian scabies, may occur in immunocompromised hosts or in conditions of severe overcrowding and poor hygiene (**Fig. 10.42**). In this form of scabies, skin lesions are crusted and widespread, resembling psoriasis, and itching is less of a feature.

Diagnosis is clinical and can be confirmed by finding the characteristic burrows in the skin and by demonstrating mites or eggs in skin scrapings. Treatment is the same as outlined above for pubic lice.

TROPICAL SEXUALLY TRANSMITTED DISEASES
Chancroid
Chancroid is an ulcerating disease of the external genitalia caused by *Haemophilus ducreyi*. Initially, after an incubation period of 3–5 days, papules form on the genitals; these soon ulcerate, with subsequent enlargement of regional lymph nodes (**Fig. 10.43**).

Autoinoculation leads to multiplication of the ulcers. These sores may heal spontaneously or they may enlarge and become locally destructive. Affected lymph nodes may develop abscesses, or buboes. Severe disease may lead to phimosis or urethral stricture.

Diagnosis may be suspected clinically and confirmed by finding Gram-negative coccobacilli in fluid from an ulcer or bubo. The organisms may appear in chains or in large groups and they may be extracellular or found within leucocytes. Culture is difficult but appropriate media are becoming more widely available.

Treatment is with erythromycin, co-trimoxazole or quinolones.

Granuloma inguinale
Granuloma inguinale, or donovanosis, is caused by a Gram-negative rod, *Calymmatobacterium granulomatis*. Although it is still endemic in southern India and

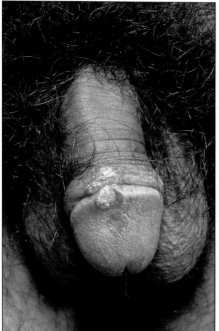

Fig. 10.43 *Chancroid ulcer in a male.*

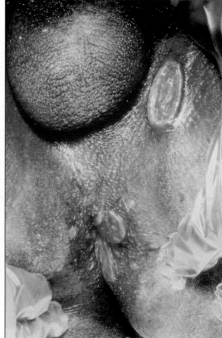

Fig. 10.44 *Granuloma inguinale in a male.*

Papua New Guinea, granuloma inguinale is becoming much less common worldwide. The disease presents with painless ulcers with a 'beefy red' base in the genital region and occasionally in the mouth (**Fig. 10.44**). Lymph node enlargement is unusual but granulomas may occur in the inguinal region and cause local swelling (pseudobuboes). The ulcers spread locally very slowly and this may lead to considerable scarring. This scarring may result in urethral, vaginal or anal stenosis.

Culture is difficult and diagnosis rests on the clinical appearances and the demonstration of the organism within large monocytes when smears are made from punch biopsy samples. Histology may also be helpful. Co-trimoxazole, erythromycin and streptomycin have all been used successfully to treat this condition.

Lymphogranuloma venereum

Lymphogranuloma venereum (LGV) is caused by three different *Chlamydia trachomatis* serovars, L1, L2 and L3. These serovars are rare in developed countries but account for up to 10% of genital ulcer disease in the tropics.

The clinical manifestations have some features in common with syphilis. Initially there is a painless genital ulcer that heals spontaneously. Women may have a purulent cervicitis at this stage. A second stage with more systemic upset then follows, characterized by malaise, headache and fever and sometimes by a mild meningitis. Erythema nodosum or a polyarthritis may occur. About one-third of patients develop large bilateral inguinal lymphadenopathy. The lymph nodes may suppurate with formation of a variable number of sinuses. A final stage of abscess formation, fistulation and rectal strictures may ensue (**Fig. 10.45**).

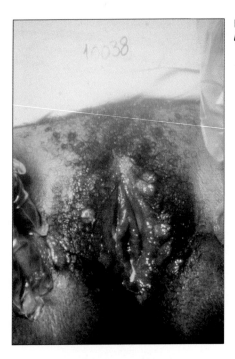

Fig. 10.45 *Ulcers secondary to lymphogranuloma venereum.*

The diagnosis is made clinically and confirmed serologically. Tetracyclines or macrolides are the treatments of choice.

REITER'S SYNDROME

Reiter's syndrome is an immune-mediated illness that sometimes follows urethritis due to *C. trachomatis* and, less frequently, occurs after a bout of bacillary dysentery. This syndrome is more common in males and is highly associated with the HLA-B27 haplotype. The most common feature is an inflammatory pauciarticular arthritis, with the ankles and knees most commonly affected. Other features are shown in **Figures 10.46** and **10.47**. Therapy is largely supportive with nonsteroidal anti-inflammatory drugs, splinting of affected joints and bed rest. There is some evidence that a 3-month course of tetracycline improves resolution of symptoms in posturethritis cases.

PELVIC INFLAMMATORY DISEASE

Pelvic inflammatory disease (PID) may complicate gonococcal or chlamydial infections in women, but other organisms, such as anaerobes, may also be involved. Ascending infection involves the fallopian tubes (salpingitis) leading to fever, pelvic pain and vaginal discharge. Clinical examination may reveal adnexal tenderness and cervical excitation.

Although PID may be suspected clinically, the features are nonspecific, so laparoscopy is often used to confirm the diagnosis (**Fig. 10.48**). Differential diagnoses include ectopic pregnancy and tubulo-ovarian abscess; therefore ultrasound plays an important role. Endocervical swabs should be taken to look for *N. gonorrhoeae* and *C. trachomatis*.

Patients with PID often need hospitalization, parenteral antibiotics and analgesia. Laparoscopic drainage of tubulo-ovarian abscesses may be required. Antibiotics should cover anaerobes as well as *N. gonorrhoeae* and *C. trachomatis*.

Clinical features of Reiter's syndrome

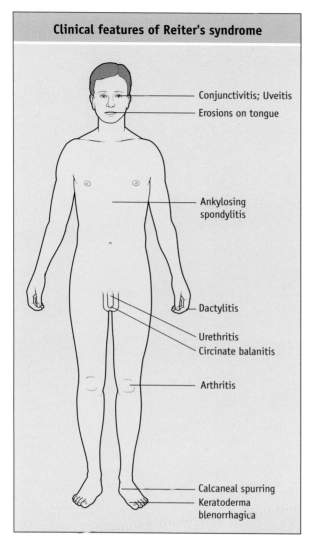

Conjunctivitis; Uveitis

Erosions on tongue

Ankylosing spondylitis

Dactylitis

Urethritis

Circinate balanitis

Arthritis

Calcaneal spurring

Keratoderma blenorrhagica

Fig. 10.46 *Clinical features of Reiter's syndrome.*

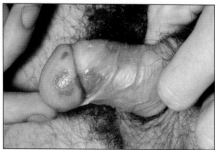

Fig. 10.47 *Circinate balanitis in Reiter's syndrome.*

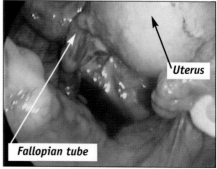

Uterus

Fallopian tube

Fig. 10.48 *Laparascopic appearances of pelvic inflammatory disease.*

chapter 11

Skin and Soft Tissue Infections

INTRODUCTION

The skin consists of a thin, avascular layer – the epidermis – overlying the much thicker dermis, which contains blood vessels, lymphatic vessels and nerves. The dermis also contains hair follicles, sebaceous glands and sweat glands. Underneath the dermis lies the subcutaneous fat, which is separated from muscle by a tough layer of fascia (**Fig. 11.1**). The skin acts as a major barrier between the host and the environment, but breaches in this barrier may lead to infection. Various infections may affect different layers of the skin.

The human skin is colonized by a variety of organisms, some of which may become invasive and cause infection in certain circumstances. Other organisms that do not normally

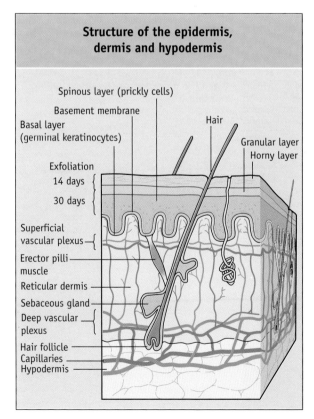

Structure of the epidermis, dermis and hypodermis

Spinous layer (prickly cells)
Basement membrane
Basal layer (germinal keratinocytes)
Hair
Granular layer
Horny layer
Exfoliation
14 days
30 days
Superficial vascular plexus
Erector pilli muscle
Reticular dermis
Sebaceous gland
Deep vascular plexus
Hair follicle
Capillaries
Hypodermis

Fig. 11.1 *Structure of normal skin.*

colonize the skin may act as pathogens if breaches in the skin occur. Coagulase-negative staphylococci are the most common skin commensals and *Staphylococcus epidermidis* is the most common of these. Other commensals include *Micrococcus* spp., coryneforms (*Corynebacterium* spp. and *Brevibacterium* spp.) and *Propionibacterium* spp. *Propionibacterium* spp. are anaerobes that normally inhabit hair follicles and sebaceous glands. *Staphylococcus aureus* may be carried on the skin by up to 20% of normal hosts, with slightly more frequent nasal carriage. Gram-negative organisms are rarely found as normal flora on the skin, although *Acinetobacter* spp. may be carried in intertriginous sites by some people.

BACTERIAL SKIN INFECTIONS

IMPETIGO

Impetigo is an infection of the epidermis. It is usually caused by *S. aureus*, but sometimes it is caused by *Streptococcus pyogenes*. Small vesicles or pustules form; these break down and weep fluid that crusts to form a golden yellow scab (**Fig. 11.2**). Sometimes impetigo presents with bullae, which are flaccid and rupture easily. This form is associated with certain strains of *S. aureus*, notably group II, phage type 71.

Impetigo is seen most often in children but is also associated with poor personal hygiene and overcrowding. Outbreaks can occur in households and in institutions. Although impetigo may heal spontaneously, antibacterial treatment accelerates healing. Topical mupirocin may be sufficient but widespread disease responds better to a systemic agent, such as flucloxacillin or clindamycin.

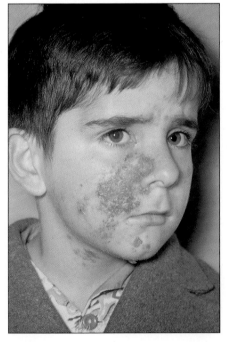

Fig. 11.2 *Impetigo, with typical yellow crusting.*

ECTHYMA

Ecthyma is similar to impetigo in that it starts with small pustules. It occurs predominantly in debilitated hosts, such as alcoholics, or following trauma. Ecthyma usually occurs on the legs and often ulcerates under the scabs. These ulcers may scar as the infection is deeper than that seen in impetigo. Systemic antistaphylococcal therapy is required.

FOLLICULITIS

Infection may occur in the hair follicles because these represent a natural break in the epidermis. There is usually a combination of occlusion of the follicle and infection, commonly with *S. aureus*. Clusters of inflamed follicles appear as red papules or pustules (**Fig. 11.3**). Antistaphylococcal therapy leads to prompt resolution.

FURUNCLES AND CARBUNCLES

If staphylococcal infection of hair follicles proceeds unabated, the dermis may be involved, leading to more extensive inflammation. When a number of furuncles coalesce, the resulting inflammatory lesion is a carbuncle, which is characterized by inflamed skin with pus coming out of hair follicles (**Fig. 11.4**). Carbuncles are seen most commonly on the back of the neck. Individual furuncles may burst and heal spontaneously but many furuncles (and all carbuncles) require incision and drainage along with systemic antistaphylococcal antibiotics.

ERYSIPELAS

This is a very superficial infection of the dermis that is almost always due to group A streptococci. Infection results in a superficial, spreading erythematous rash with well-demarcated edges (**Fig. 11.5**). It occurs most frequently on the face; it is sometimes seen on the legs. There are often systemic features such as fever and rigors. The treatment of choice is benzylpenicillin or clindamycin.

CELLULITIS

This is a spreading infection of the deeper dermis and subcutaneous fat; the depth of inflammation differentiates it from erysipelas. The usual micro-organisms implicated are group A streptococci and *S. aureus*, but Gram-negative aerobes and anaerobes may sometimes be involved. Most cases involve the lower limbs (**Fig. 11.6**). Cellulitis may follow trivial injuries to the skin or it may result from breaches in the skin resulting from tinea infections or eczema. Sometimes more obvious damage, such as puncture wounds or animal

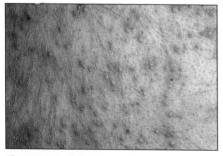

Fig. 11.3 *Inflamed hair follicles in folliculitis.*

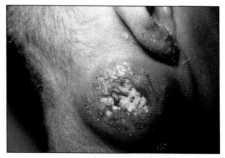

Fig. 11.4 *A typical carbuncle.*

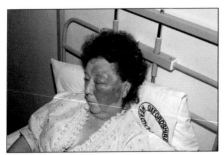

Fig. 11.5 *Well-demarcated infection in facial erysipelas.*

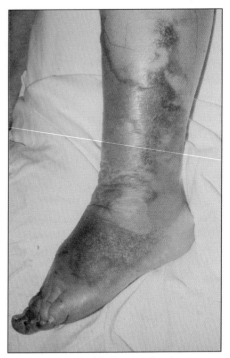

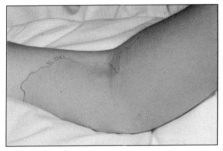

Fig. 11.7 *Cellulitis of the arm following a cat scratch.*

Fig. 11.6 *Marked inflammation in cellulitis.*

bites, may result in cellulitis (**Fig. 11.7**). Patients with ischaemic legs, varicose ulcers, lymphoedema and diabetes mellitus are all at increased risk of cellulitis.

The diagnosis of cellulitis is almost entirely clinical. Blood cultures are rarely positive, skin swabs are useless and skin biopsies or tissue aspirates rarely yield positive cultures. However, if there is an obvious collection of pus or any blisters, these should be cultured.

Treatment should be directed at Gram-positive cocci, primarily at *S. aureus* and streptococci. Anaerobic cover should be added if there are leg ulcers or if the patient has diabetes mellitus. Elevation of the limb and subcutaneous heparin are useful adjunctive measures.

UNUSUAL INFECTIONS
Anthrax
Anthrax is a rare condition that is caused by *Bacillus anthracis*. It most commonly affects the skin and usually results in a so-called malignant pustule. The infection results from the inoculation of bacterial spores into skin abrasions and is most often acquired occupationally from the hides of infected animals. A few days after inoculation a papule forms; this develops into a vesicle, which, in turn, ulcerates. There is often local oedema and painful regional lymphadenopathy. The necrotic centre of the ulcer forms an eschar (**Fig. 11.8**). Systemic features are common and bacteraemia may result in death.

The diagnosis may be suspected clinically and confirmed by finding Gram-positive bacilli in the ulcer fluid or tissues (**Fig. 11.9**) and culturing the organism. Benzylpenicillin is the treatment of choice.

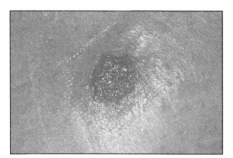

Fig. 11.8 *Necrotic skin lesion in cutaneous anthrax.*

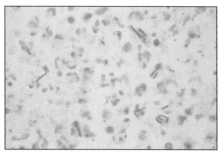

Fig. 11.9 *Histology of anthrax lesion showing Gram-positive rods.*

Erysipeloid

Erysipeloid is caused by a facultative anaerobic Gram-positive bacillus, *Erysipelothrix rhusiopathiae*. The most common risk factor is contact with infected animals, particularly pigs, so veterinary surgeons, farmers and butchers may be affected. The fingers and hands are the most commonly involved sites from direct inoculation, and dark, purplish lesions and swelling of the digits often develop (**Fig. 11.10**). Rarely, sepsis may ensue. The skin disease responds to penicillin.

Pyoderma gangrenosum

Pyoderma gangrenosum is a condition of unknown aetiology. It is sometimes seen in association with rheumatoid arthritis or inflammatory bowel disease, but it may occur on its own. Pyoderma gangrenosum may start as a small vesicle that ulcerates. The ulcer slowly expands with a necrotic base and a characteristic violaceous edge with surrounding erythema (**Fig. 11.11**). It may have the appearance of an infected wound. However, samples from the ulcer or its edge are always sterile and antibiotic therapy has no effect on the disease process. This condition also demonstrates the phenomenon of pathergy, in that it may occur at sites of skin trauma, including operative wounds or venepuncture sites. Healing is effected by immunosuppression with corticosteroids and, sometimes, cyclosporin. Other drugs that have been used include dapsone and minocycline.

Necrotizing fasciitis

Necrotizing fasciitis is a rapidly spreading destructive infection of the subcutaneous fat and superficial fascia. Group A streptococci are often involved, usually acting synergistically with anaerobic organisms. Necrotizing fasciitis usually follows an injury, either a trivial wound or some form of (often minor) surgery. Superficially it may resemble cellulitis but it

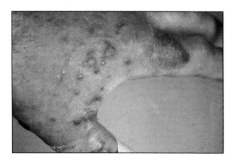

Fig. 11.10 *Infected fingers in erysipeloid.*

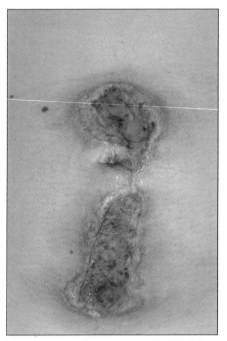

Fig. 11.11 *Pyoderma gangrenosum with typical violaceous ulcer border.*

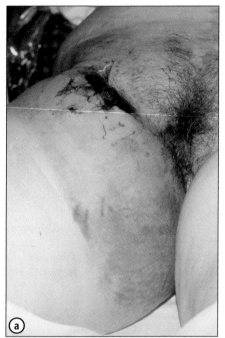

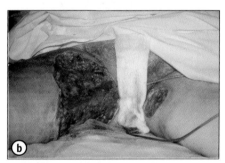

Fig. 11.12 *Necrotizing fasciitis: (a) necrotic wound following coronary angiography with subcutaneous necrosis in thigh appearing as bruising; (b) same patient showing extent of debridement of necrotic tissues at operation.*

responds poorly to antibiotic therapy and progresses rapidly, and the tissues often appear bruised owing to the subcutaneous necrosis (**Fig 11.12**). Characteristically, the affected tissues are exquisitely painful, quite unlike the situation in cellulitis. Systemic features of toxicity are common and shock is a frequent problem.

The diagnosis may be suspected clinically and is confirmed by surgical exploration: CT or MRI scanning may show obvious abnormalities of the soft tissues. (**Fig. 11.13**). Successful treatment requires aggressive surgical debridement, broad-spectrum antibiotics and intensive supportive care.

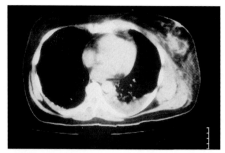

Fig. 11.13 *CT scan of necrotic tissue in necrotizing fasciitis.*

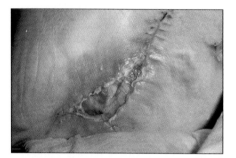

Fig. 11.15 *Inflamed wound with a purulent centre.*

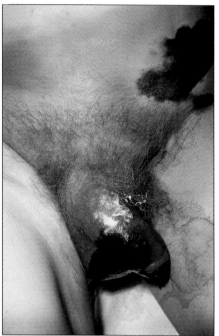

Fig. 11.14 *Fourniere's gangrene in a patient with diabetes mellitus.*

Fourniere's gangrene

Fourniere's gangrene is a term used to describe a form of necrotizing fasciitis that affects the male genitalia. Although it may occur spontaneously, it most frequently occurs in debilitated hospitalized men over the age of 50 years. Diabetes mellitus is a predisposing condition. The scrotum, penis and anterior abdominal wall may all be involved in the process (**Fig. 11.14**). There is usually a mixture of organisms involved, many of bowel origin. Surgical debridement and broad-spectrum antibiotics with good anaerobic cover are required.

Wound infections

Before the days of prophylactic antibiotic therapy, surgical wound infection was a major problem. Though less common now, wound infections are still seen, particularly in debilitated or immunosuppressed patients. The causative organisms are usually *S. aureus* and other skin flora. The infected wound becomes reddened and there may be pain and a spreading cellulitis (**Fig. 11.15**). Systemic features other than fever are unusual. In severe cases the surgical wound may dehisce. Treatment consists of systemic antibiotics; debridement or drainage of pus may also be required.

Gas gangrene

Gas gangrene is an anaerobic infection that is usually due to *Clostridium perfringens*. It is rare but may follow trauma involving contaminated wounds. The infection involves skin, subcutaneous tissues and muscle and is characterized by severe systemic upset, gas formation in the affected tissues and an unpleasant odour (**Fig. 11.16**). Shock and other problems, such

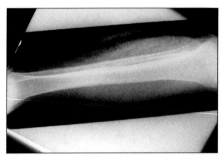

Fig. 11.16 *Gas in tissues on plain X-ray.*

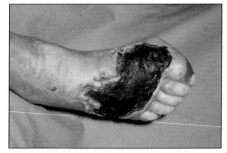

Fig. 11.17 *Infected burn wound.*

as disseminated intravascular coagulation, are common. There is a high mortality. Aggressive surgical management and high doses of parenteral antibiotics are needed.

Burns

Burns, particularly full-thickness burns, destroy the integrity of the skin as a barrier and leave large areas of the subcutaneous tissues exposed to the risk of infection. Affected tissue may change colour or the surrounding unburned skin may become oedematous and painful (**Fig. 11.17**). Systemic symptoms, such as fever and tachycardia, may indicate the onset of infection in these patients. *Pseudomonas aeruginosa* and *S. aureus* are the most common bacteria involved in invasive infections of burns patients. Other organisms, such as fungi and viruses, may also be implicated in some cases.

Infections in burns cases are often prevented now by using a combination of meticulous wound toilet, early skin coverage and topical antibacterial agents. Signs of invasive infection should be sought and promptly treated with appropriate parenteral antibiotics.

Ulcers

Skin ulcers may occasionally be due to specific infections but they are more commonly caused by other means; however, they may become colonized with bacteria and sometimes become secondarily infected. Skin necrosis secondary to pressure (pressure sores or decubitus ulcers) may occur, particularly in elderly, ill patients with fragile skin or in paraplegic patients who lack sensation in pressure areas. Pressure sores usually become colonized with a mixture of aerobic and anaerobic bacteria and can act as a source of systemic sepsis in debilitated patients. This is often preceded by cellulitis around the pressure sore (**Fig. 11.18**).

Ulcers secondary to neuropathy are most commonly seen in the feet of people with diabetes mellitus. Like decubitus ulcers, these neuropathic ulcers usually contain a mixture of bacteria. Soft tissue infection in this setting may lead to osteomyelitis locally but occasionally goes on to cause systemic sepsis.

Poor vascular supply to the skin is a feature of venous insufficiency that usually affects the lower extremities. Venous ulcers may result spontaneously or after minor trauma. These ulcers rapidly become colonized, usually with *S. aureus* and sometimes with Gram-negative bacilli. Antibiotic treatment is only warranted if there is associated cellulitis. Ischaemic ulcers in the feet may also result from peripheral arterial disease, and *S. aureus* is a common colonizer.

Soft tissue infection related to intravenous drug usage

Intravenous drug users frequently introduce bacteria into normally sterile sites. Although the biggest danger is infective endocarditis, soft tissue infections are a more frequent

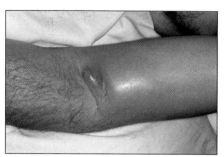

Fig. 11.19 *Abscess in an intravenous drug user.*

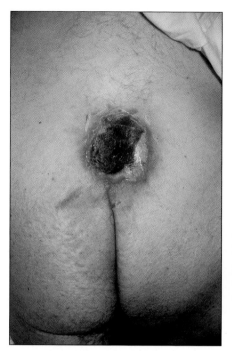

Fig. 11.18 *Infected pressure area wound.*

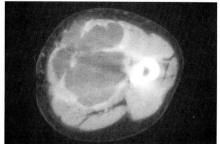

Fig. 11.20 *Thigh abscess due to Streptococcus milleri in an intravenous drug user (CT scan).*

problem. Abscesses at the site of injection may occur and cause considerable soft tissue damage (**Fig. 11.19**). Injections may also lead to intramuscular abscesses in intravenous drug users who have inaccessible veins (**Fig. 11.20**). Infections in intravenous drug users are usually due either to *S. aureus* or to bacteria that are commonly found in the mouth, such as streptococci. Treatment is with antibiotics; some form of surgical drainage or debridement is also usually needed.

MUSCLE INFECTIONS

BACTERIAL INFECTIONS

Abscesses

The psoas muscle is one of the most common muscles involved in pyogenic infection. A psoas abscess may present with just a fever but there may also be local pain or tenderness. In addition, there may be limitation of hip movement with accentuation of pain when the hip is extended and the inflamed psoas muscle is stretched. Such abscesses may occur spontaneously following a transient bacteraemia, when the usual cause is *S. aureus*, or they may be involved in local intra-abdominal sepsis (**Fig. 11.21**). This may occur in Crohn's disease, for example, when the causative organisms are a mixture of aerobic and anaerobic bowel flora. Rarely, a psoas abscess (or an abscess in another muscle) may be due to tuberculosis.

Psoas abscesses usually require some form of drainage procedure in addition to antibiotics. This is usually done percutaneously with computed tomography guidance, but open drainage is sometimes required.

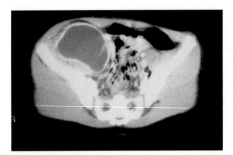

Fig. 11.21 *Psoas abscess due to Staphylococcus aureus.*

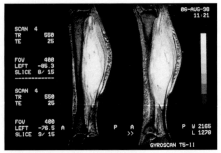

Fig. 11.22 *MRI scan showing pyomyositis in the leg.*

Myositis

Bacterial myositis is rare in developed countries but is still relatively common in the tropics, although the reasons for this difference are poorly understood. Most cases are due to *S. aureus*. Usually several muscle groups are involved, but the quadriceps is the most frequently affected. The patients are usually young men who present with muscle pain that is followed some time later by fever and localized swelling. The affected muscles initially have a woody induration and later become fluctuant as the deep abscess 'ripens'.

Ultrasound can locate the intramuscular abscesses but blind needle aspiration is often used diagnostically in the tropics; the aspirated pus is reddish-pink owing to necrotic muscle (**Fig. 11.22**). Treatment is with surgical debridement and antistaphylococcal antibiotics.

VIRAL MYOSITIS

Myositis can occasionally complicate viral infections. In children with influenza, myositis may occur towards the end of the illness. There is pain on walking, the muscles are tender and the creatine kinase level is elevated. Myoglobinuria does not occur and the disease runs a benign course with complete recovery, usually within 1 week. A more severe myositis occurs rarely in adults after influenza or enteroviral infections. In adults, myoglobinuria may lead to acute renal failure.

PARASITIC INFECTIONS

A variety of parasites may involve the muscles (**Fig. 11.23**). Often these are asymptomatic but sometimes an overt myositis occurs.

Fig. 11.23 *Parasites that may involve muscle.*

Parasites that may involve muscle
Trichinella spiralis
Taenia solium (cysticerca)
Toxocara canis
Toxoplasma gondii
Trypanosoma cruzi

FUNGAL SKIN INFECTIONS

CANDIDAL INFECTIONS

Candida albicans is part of the normal flora of the skin, mucosae and bowel and rarely causes infection. However, skin infections may follow broad-spectrum antibiotic therapy or occur in compromised hosts, such as those with diabetes mellitus or those receiving corticosteroids. Infection is most common in the moist, warm folds of skin in the axillae, under the breasts, in the natal cleft and between rolls of fat in obese people (**Fig. 11.24**). The skin is reddened and itchy and there may be a whitish, sticky exudate. Sometimes infections of the nail fold (paronychia) occur and may go on to involve the nail bed.

Diagnosis is usually easy clinically and can be confirmed by demonstrating budding yeasts from swabs of affected areas. Treatment with topical antifungal agents, such as miconazole, is usually successful, particularly if underlying risk factors are improved. Extensive disease may require systemic therapy with fluconazole or itraconazole.

DERMATOPHYTE INFECTIONS

Most superficial fungal skin infections are caused by dermatophytes that have a predilection for keratin. These ubiquitous fungi are grouped into three main genera: *Trichophyton*, *Microsporum* and *Epidermophyton*. Hair, nails and the stratum corneum of the skin are the affected tissues; all of these tissues share the features of being non-viable and frequently shed from the body.

Tinea capitis

Sometimes called scalp ringworm, tinea capitis is mainly a disease of children. *Trichophyton* spp. are the most common causes of this condition. The fungi infect the hair shaft at any stage of hair growth and can lead to a variety of clinical presentations. The most common is the development of patchy hair loss with little in the way of skin inflammation (**Fig. 11.25**). Sometimes there may be scaling that resembles seborrhoeic dermatitis. Rarely there may be severe inflammation.

Diagnosis is by demonstrating the fungus by potassium hydroxide examination of hairs from the affected area. Cultures should be set up on Sabouraud agar. Treatment is with griseofulvin, which needs to be given for several weeks. Recently, terbinafine has become more widely used for this condition.

Tinea corporis

Any of the dermatophyte species may infect the stratum corneum of the skin. Although children are often infected, any age group may be affected. Infection is transmitted from another affected person or from animals. The skin lesions start as small papules that

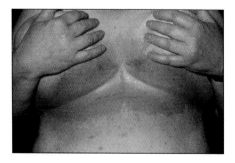

Fig. 11.24 *Intertrigo caused by* Candida albicans.

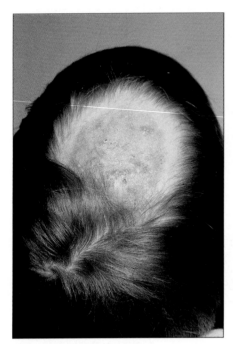

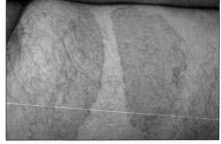

Fig. 11.26 *Tinea corporis or ringworm.*

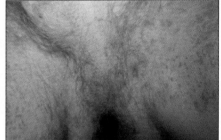

Fig. 11.25 *Scalp ringworm.*

Fig. 11.27 *Tinea cruris.*

subsequently enlarge outwards. This leads to itchy patches of inflammation with raised, scaly red edges and a relatively clear central area (**Fig. 11.26**). Occasionally the skin lesions can be vesicular or remain as multiple red papules.

The diagnosis is clinical and confirmed by potassium hydroxide examination and culture. Topical antifungals such as miconazole are often adequate, but extensive disease may require systemic therapy. Griseofulvin has been the mainstay of treatment but itraconazole may now be a better choice.

Tinea cruris

Dermatophyte infections of the groin and perineum are much more common in men than in women. The pruritic rash usually has a well-defined margin (**Fig. 11.27**). Topical antifungal treatment, sometimes with initial topical corticosteroids for the inflammatory component, usually work. Systemic treatment may be needed, particularly in patients with diabetes mellitus or immunocompromised patients.

Tinea pedis

Athlete's foot, or tinea pedis, is one of the most common fungal infections in the world. The most common cause is *Trichophyton rubrum* but other species of dermatophyte may also be involved. Infections often begin in the web of skin between the toes, with fungal growth encouraged by humidity and warmth. Tinea pedis may present with an itchy, red rash or there may be little inflammation but, instead, hyperkeratosis. The latter is more common in chronic infections and may involve the soles of the feet. This condition may be complicated by secondary bacterial infection, which requires permanganate soaks and systemic antibiotics (**Fig. 11.28**). Uncomplicated tinea pedis may be treated with topical antifungal creams or, if chronic, with systemic antifungal agents.

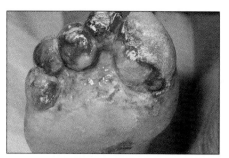

Fig. 11.28 *Pseudomonal secondary infection in athlete's foot.*

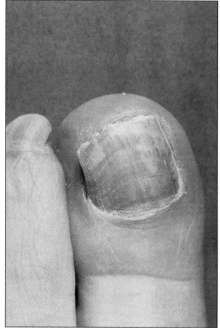

Fig. 11.29 *Onychomycosis.*

Onychomycosis

Trichophyton spp. are usually the only dermatophytes that infect the nail bed or nail plate. Onychomycosis is largely a disease of adults and is usually seen in conjunction with tinea pedis and, sometimes, the equivalent condition in the hand, tinea manuum. Other fungi, such as *Candida* spp., may also cause onychomycosis.

The nails become discoloured and distorted and may be quite friable (**Fig. 11.29**). Potassium hydroxide examination and fungal culture help to differentiate onychomycosis from other conditions such as psoriatic inflammation of the nails. Griseofulvin has long been used to treat onychomycosis but terbinafine is now the treatment of choice. Itraconazole can also be used for dermatophyte infections and is usually the best treatment for nondermaphyte nail infections.

VIRAL INFECTIONS OF THE SKIN

HERPESVIRUS INFECTIONS

Herpes simplex virus

Although herpes simplex virus (HSV) commonly affects the mucosae of the mouth and genitals, it can also affect the skin (**Fig. 11.30**). Like all herpesviruses, HSV exhibits latency and may be reactivated after a primary infection, leading to cold sores. Spread by direct contact occurs and may involve extensive areas of skin. This is more likely if the skin is abnormal, as it is in eczema. The florid spread of HSV under these circumstances is called eczema herpeticum. (**Fig. 11.31**). Herpetic whitlows are HSV infections of the hand that arise after contact with infected saliva (**Fig. 11.32**).

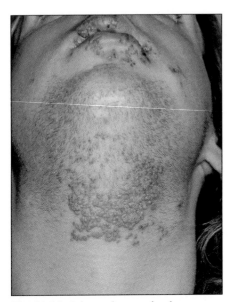

Fig. 11.30 *Primary herpes simplex infection.*

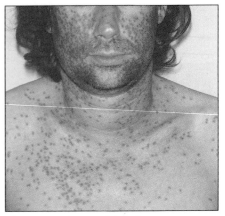

Fig. 11.31 *Eczema herpeticum.*

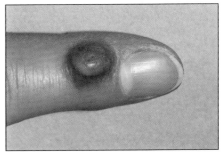

Fig. 11.32 *Herpetic whitlow.*

Diagnosis is often easy clinically but can be confirmed by culturing HSV from skin lesions or demonstrating a herpesvirus by electron microscopy. Most infections are self-limiting but antiviral drugs such as aciclovir accelerate healing, though they do not influence the rates of recurrence.

Varicella-zoster virus

Varicella-zoster virus (VZV) causes chickenpox in previously unexposed people. The typical rash occurs 2–3 weeks after infection and usually follows a short prodrome of malaise and fever. Chickenpox appears as crops of vesicles with erythematous bases that are centrally distributed on the trunk and head before spreading to the limbs. New crops may appear for up to 1 week. The vesicles usually turn into pustules; these may become haemorrhagic and they eventually scab over (**Fig. 11.33**). Adults are generally more severely ill than children with chickenpox and have a greater risk of pneumonitis and encephalitis.

Chickenpox is usually obvious clinically but it can be confirmed by electron microscopy of vesicle fluid, by culture or by serology. Children recover uneventfully but treatment with systemic antiviral agents, such as aciclovir, is used in adults, neonates and immunocompromised patients.

Shingles, or herpes zoster, is due to reactivation of latent VZV in people who have had chickenpox at some time in the past. The virus is present in dorsal root ganglia and when reactivated it tracks down the sensory nerves to cause skin lesions (vesicles) in the dermatome served by that nerve (**Figs. 11.34** and **11.35**). The lesions are often painful and

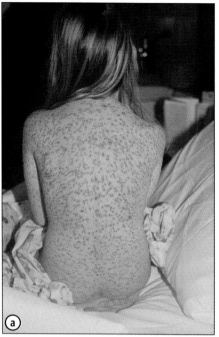

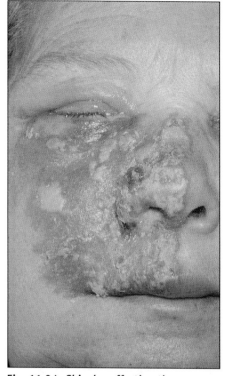

Fig. 11.34 *Shingles affecting the maxillary division of the right fifth cranial nerve.*

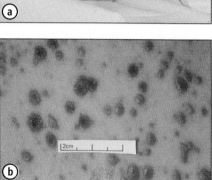

Fig. 11.33 *(a) and (b) Chickenpox.*

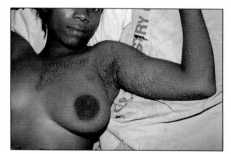

Fig. 11.35 *Acute shingles affecting a thoracic dermatome (T1).*

there may be systemic upset. Sometimes there is viral replication within the meninges, leading to a lymphocytic meningitis.

Multidermatomal involvement, bilateral shingles and disseminated shingles are all rare but may occur in immunocompromised hosts. Shingles may be complicated by secondary bacterial infection. A small number of patients go on to develop postherpetic neuralgia, which can be quite debilitating.

Most cases of shingles resolve spontaneously. Systemic antiviral therapy limits acute pain and improves the rate of healing. The evidence that treatment reduces postherpetic neuralgia is less convincing.

ENTEROVIRUS INFECTIONS

Enteroviral infections, especially those due to echoviruses and Coxsackieviruses, frequently involve the skin. Most commonly there is a fine erythematous macular rash and this is more common in children than adults. Some Coxsackievirus types, such as A16, are associated with small vesicles with a red margin. These lesions appear on the hands, feet and in the oral cavity; hence the name of the resulting disease, hand, foot and mouth disease (**Figs. 11.36** and **11.37**).

POXVIRUSES

Molluscum contagiosum

Molluscum contagiosum is spread by close human contact and results in small, umbilicated skin lesions. The disease is benign and the lesions persist for a few weeks and then disappear spontaneously. In people infected with HIV, the lesions may not clear and some may become very large (**Fig. 11.38**). Intralesional liquid nitrogen may speed regression.

Orf

Orf is transmitted to humans from infected lambs and goats and is thus an occupational hazard of farmers and veterinary surgeons. The skin lesions start as papules and then enlarge, often becoming haemorrhagic pustules. Most of the pustules occur on the hands but the virus can be autoinoculated to other sites (**Fig. 11.39**). The patient is systemically

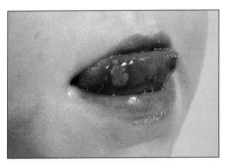

Fig. 11.36 *Oral lesions in hand, foot and mouth disease.*

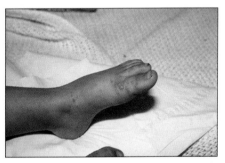

Fig. 11.37 *Skin vesicles in hand, foot and mouth disease.*

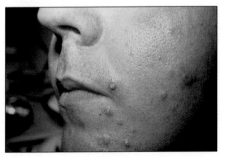

Fig. 11.38 *Umbilicated lesions of molluscum contagiosum.*

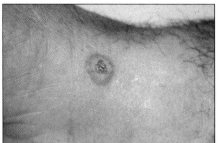

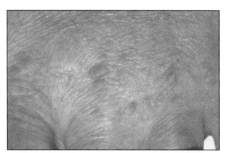

Fig. 11.39 *Orf lesion on a farmer's arm.*   Fig. 11.40 *Common warts on the fingers.*

well and after a few days the pustules ulcerate, scab over and heal spontaneously. The diagnosis is usually made on clinical grounds, but fluid from the pustules will reveal poxviruses if examined by electron microscopy.

Warts

In addition to causing genital warts (condylomata acuminata), human papilloma viruses (HPVs) also cause warts elsewhere. These deoxyribonucleic acid (DNA) viruses are spread by close human contact and are most common in older children and teenagers. They are also frequently seen in solid organ transplant recipients and, sometimes, in patients with acquired immunodeficiency syndrome (AIDS).

Common warts, usually due to HPV type 2 (HPV-2), are rough, keratinized papules that can occur anywhere but are most often found on the hands (**Fig. 11.40**). They contain thrombosed capillaries; therefore if the warts are pared with a knife the capillaries appear as small dark dots. Deeper paring may cause pinpoint bleeding. There are usually multiple warts and they are asymptomatic.

Plantar warts occur on the soles of the feet, usually in children, and grow inwards (**Fig. 11.41**). These warts, caused by HPV type 1 (HPV-1), are usually single and can be painful.

Flat, or planar warts, form very small, flat papules in the skin and are usually multiple. Caused by HPV type 3 (HPV-3), they are most frequently seen on the face and hands.

Except in immunocompromised patients, warts regress spontaneously and rarely cause any problems. There is no premalignant potential. However, if the warts are cosmetically unacceptable or are painful, patients may demand treatment. Most treatments involve the topical application of substances such as salicylic acid, formaldehyde, podophyllin or liquid nitrogen. Recurrence is common.

VIRAL EXANTHEMS

Measles (rubeola)

The measles virus is a paramyxovirus and is very contagious. After an incubation period of 10–14 days, there is a fever, upper respiratory tract symptoms, conjunctivitis and malaise. The rash starts 3 or 4 days later, usually at the height of the fever, and may be preceded by Koplik spots (**Fig. 11.42**) appearing on the buccal mucosa. The measles rash starts behind the ears and descends over the body surface, sparing the palms and soles (**Fig. 11.43**). The rash initially consists of discrete pink macules that blanche on pressure, but it soon coalesces and darkens to a coppery colour; the whole process lasts about 1 week. There may be some desquamation after this.

171

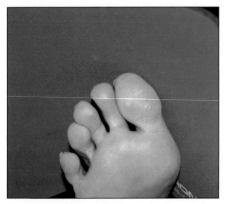

Fig. 11.41 *Plantar warts.*

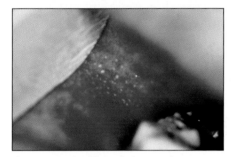

Fig. 11.42 *Koplik spots in measles.*

Fig. 11.43 *Typical measles rash.*

Children look and feel miserable with measles but soon recover. Adults may be more ill. Immunocompromised patients may get a severe rash and are at increased risk of complications. In children, the most common complications are otitis media and secondary bacterial pneumonia. Rarely, an acute encephalitis or subacute sclerosing panencephalitis (SSPE) may ensue. Measles in pregnant women does not result in congenital disease but may increase the risk of miscarriage.

The diagnosis of measles is a clinical one but can be confirmed by viral isolation from nasopharyngeal secretions or by using a specific enzyme-linked immunosorbent assay to measure antibody or detect an antibody rise in paired sera. Treatment is supportive and the disease is becoming less common as a result of widespread use of a live, attenuated measles virus vaccine.

Rubella

Rubella virus is a single stranded ribonucleic acid virus, which, unlike the measles virus, produces a rather mild disease. The virus is spread by respiratory droplets with clinical features appearing about 14–21 days after infection. Most cases are mild and some are asymptomatic. Children usually develop an erythematous macular rash that first appears on the face and then spreads to the rest of the body. They frequently have cervical lymphadenopathy and mild conjunctivitis (**Fig. 11.44**). Adults sometimes develop a rash but, more commonly, arthralgia and arthritis are the presenting features. Clinical diagnosis is unreliable and diagnosis thus depends on finding specific IgM antibodies in the serum or a rise in IgG levels over time. There are no long-term sequelae of rubella.

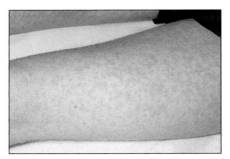

Fig. 11.44 *Rubella rash.*

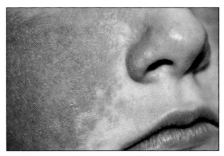

Fig. 11.45 *'Slapped cheeks' appearance of acute parvovirus infection.*

Congenital rubella syndrome occurs in the children of mothers infected during pregnancy. The biggest risk is during the first trimester; infections in the third trimester rarely lead to problems. Some of the clinical features of congenital infection are transient, but many children have developmental abnormalities and some have the classical triad of patent ductus arteriosus, cataracts and neural deafness.

Erythema infectiosum

Erythema infectiosum, or fifth disease, is a benign disease of childhood caused by parvovirus B19, a single-stranded DNA virus. It is highly infectious and is spread by respiratory droplets. The affected child is usually very well, sometimes with a macular rash, but often presents with bright red cheeks, hence the other name for this disease, 'slapped cheek syndrome' (**Fig. 11.45**). Adults often develop a macular, erythematous rash and may develop an acute polyarthropathy. Hands, knees and feet are the most frequently affected joints, usually with a symmetrical distribution.

This virus is easily dealt with by the normal host but, because it is trophic for red blood cell precursors, it may cause aplastic crises in patients with sickle cell disease. Maternal infection in the second trimester may lead to hydrops fetalis.

Parvovirus infections are diagnosed serologically, based either on a positive IgM test or a rise in IgG antibodies over time.

Roseola

Sometimes referred to as 'sixth disease', roseola, or exanthem subitum, is caused by human herpes virus (HHV-6). Typically, about 10 days after infection, the affected child presents with a rash on its back and neck; the rash subsequently spreads to the chest and limbs but the face and feet are spared. The rash is accompanied by high fever, lymphadenopathy and coryzal symptoms. Up to 10% of children may experience a febrile seizure.

The disease is self-limiting and has no sequelae. The rash lasts about 48–72 hours. The diagnosis is made serologically.

Kawasaki disease

Kawasaki disease, or mucocutaneous lymph node syndrome, is a disease of childhood of unknown aetiology. It may present like an infection and be mistaken for a viral exanthem. Toddlers are most commonly affected. The illness starts with high fevers, which are soon followed by an erythematous rash, usually in association with oedema of the hands and feet (**Fig. 11.46**). The oral cavity and tongue may become bright red with inflammation, and

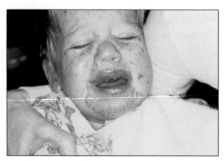 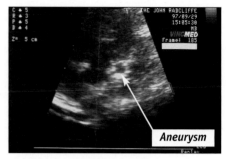

Fig. 11.46 *Skin appearances in Kawasaki sydrome.*

Fig. 11.47 *Coronary artery aneurysm in Kawasaki syndrome.*

there may be conjunctival injection. There is usually cervical lymphadenopathy. After 5–7 days the rash on the hands and feet begins to fade, although it may persist elsewhere, and there is often desquamation at the extremities.

The systemic features become predominant at this stage; these are characterized by an arteritis. In severe cases, the coronary arteries are involved and may become aneurysmal, sometimes causing myocardial ischaemia and myocardial infarction.

There are no diagnostic tests, but raised inflammatory markers and elevated platelet counts are characteristic. Echocardiography may detect coronary artery aneurysms (**Fig. 11.47**). Trials have shown that Kawasaki disease responds well to intravenous immunoglobulin therapy and oral aspirin.

chapter 12

Bone and Joint Infections

INTRODUCTION

Bone is a dynamic tissue – through osteoclast and osteoblast activity, it is capable of remarkable growth and remodelling. Bone growth before puberty occurs at the end of the metaphysis at the epiphyseal growth plate. This growth plate gets its blood supply via the metaphysis from what are essentially end-arterioles. Capillaries from the arterioles form loops in the epiphyseal growth plate and venous blood returns through sluggishly flowing sinuses (**Fig. 12.1**). With increasing age the epiphysis, which is initially almost entirely made of cartilage, becomes ossified and fuses with the metaphysis. The blood supply of the epiphyseal plate means that if infection and inflammation develop there, blockage of the arterioles may occur, with subsequent necrosis. This may partly explain the increased incidence of acute bone infection in prepubertal children.

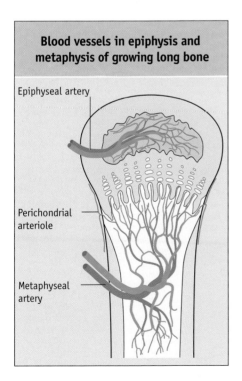

Blood vessels in epiphysis and metaphysis of growing long bone

Epiphyseal artery

Perichondrial arteriole

Metaphyseal artery

Fig. 12.1 *Blood vessels in the epiphysis and metaphysis.*

OSTEOMYELITIS

Infection of the bone may involve:
- the medullary cavity;
- the cortical (or hard) bone; or
- the periosteum.

Frequently, all three components are involved.

Infection leads to inflammation in the bone and, as pressure builds within the rigid bone, thrombosis of local vessels occurs with subsequent necrosis of bone. The relatively avascular site of infection allows organisms to proliferate and be relatively protected from host defences. Eventually islands of dead bone (sequestra) may form and these can act as niduses for continued infection and be relatively inaccessible to antimicrobial agents (**Fig. 12.2**). Unchecked, the infection may spread through the bone, either into a joint or through the periosteum into the soft tissues, sometimes with the subsequent formation of a sinus tract. Osteomyelitis is usually caused by bacteria (**Fig. 12.3**) and is either acute or chronic. It may arise in one of three ways:
- by haematogenous spread;
- from a contiguous source; or
- because of vascular insufficiency.

HAEMATOGENOUS OSTEOMYELITIS

Most cases of childhood osteomyelitis, and some cases in adults, are acute and result from a bacteraemia. *Staphylococcus aureus* is the most commonly implicated bacteria but coagulase-negative staphylococci and streptococci are sometimes involved. *Haemophilus*

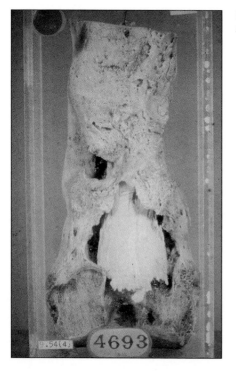

Fig. 12.2 *Museum specimen showing a sequestrum in chronic osteomyelitis.*

Organisms causing osteomyelitis in children and adults

Children	Adults
Staphylococcus aureus	*Staphylococcus aureus*
Group B streptococci	Enterobacteriaceae
Escherichia coli	Bacteroides spp., especially in patients with diabetes mellitus (in whom other anaerobes may also cause osteomyelitis)
Salmonella spp. (in patients with sickle cell disease)	*Pasteurella multocida* (transmitted by animal bites)
Haemophilus influenzae	*Brucella melitensis* (osteomyelitis is usually vertebral)
Eikenella corrodens	*Mycobacterium tuberculosis*
	Coagulase-negative staphylococcus (causes device-related osteomyelitis)

Fig. 12.3 *Organisms causing osteomyelitis in children and adults.*

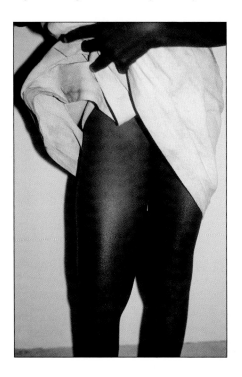

Fig. 12.4 *Acute haematogenous osteomyelitis of the femur.*

influenzae type b used to be a relatively common cause of osteomyelitis in childhood but it is rapidly disappearing following successful immunization programmes.

In acute childhood osteomyelitis there are often fever and rigors in association with the initial bacteraemia, with local pain and swelling occurring some time later (**Fig. 12.4**). There may be loss of function of the affected limb owing to pain. Adults may have more subtle symptoms with mild fever and malaise and poor localization of signs.

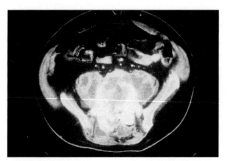

Fig. 12.5 *Pelvic abscess involving a vertebral body.*

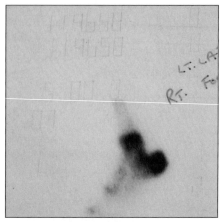

Fig. 12.6 *Bone scan with hot spot at an area of osteomyelitis.*

OSTEOMYELITIS SECONDARY TO A CONTIGUOUS SOURCE

Infection in adjacent tissue may extend to involve the bone (**Fig. 12.5**); for example:

- the bones of the pelvis may become involved as a result of intra-abdominal infection;
- the sacrum may be involved if pressure sores are deep and infected; and
- fractures may become infected as a result of contaminated wounds.

An increasingly common problem is infection following the insertion of a prosthetic joint. In these settings a variety of organisms may be involved. Both coagulase-positive and coagulase-negative staphylococci are still important but Enterobacteriaceae, *Pseudomonas* spp. and anaerobes are increasingly seen in this setting.

Most cases of osteomyelitis in this category occur in adults. Usually the symptoms and signs of the local infection are obvious, although the bone involvement may not be apparent. In these cases osteomyelitis should be sought by probing the wound, aspirating deep tissue samples or by surgical exploration.

OSTEOMYELITIS SECONDARY TO VASCULAR INSUFFICIENCY

Arterial insufficiency due to peripheral vascular disease or diabetes mellitus (or both) compromises the viability of skin and bone and increases the risk of infection. Ulcers may occur and become infected, with infection tracking down to bone. Associated neuropathy means that such infections may be relatively painless. A large variety of organisms may cause infection in this setting and polymicrobial osteomyelitis is not unusual.

DIAGNOSIS OF OSTEOMYELITIS

Just as the clinical features can be variable, indirect evidence of inflammation is not invariably present. There may be a leucocytosis or inflammatory markers such as the erythrocyte sedimentation rate (ESR) or C-reactive protein (CRP) may be elevated. Blood cultures are often positive in acute haematogenous osteomyelitis in children but are rarely positive in other types of osteomyelitis. Changes on plain X-rays take time to develop so that films may be normal during the acute phase of infection. Radioisotope scans (**Fig. 12.6**) can show areas of increased osteoclast activity at a very early stage when plain X-rays are

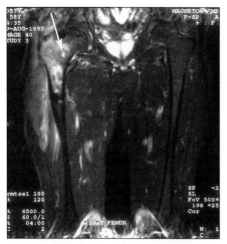

Fig. 12.7 *MRI scan showing increased signal in a femur with osteomyelitis.*

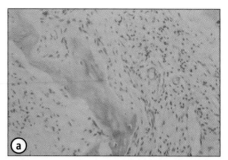

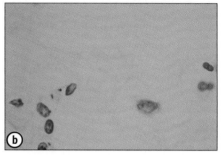

Fig. 12.8 *Histology in osteomyelitis: (a) Bone biopsy showing acute inflammatory cells; (b) Gram stain of biopsy material showing Gram-positive cocci (*Staphylococcus aureus*).*

normal. Increasingly, computed tomography (CT) scans and magnetic resonance imaging (MRI) scans are being used. Magnetic resonance imaging may show very early changes of inflammation in the medullary cavity (**Fig. 12.7**). However, MRI may be difficult to interpret after surgery or if there has been previous infection, because the changes may take a long time to resolve.

The bacteriological diagnosis can be determined by sampling the affected bone. In acute osteomyelitis this may involve the sampling of pus from an intramedullary abscess by drilling through the bone. Frequently, samples for culture are obtained by percutaneous bone biopsy using an image intensifier or CT scan. Histology may be useful but it rarely gives an aetiological diagnosis (**Fig. 12.8**). Obtaining reliable tissue samples for culture is critical to the successful management of osteomyelitis. However, if acute osteomyelitis is suspected clinically, treatment should be started empirically while the results of cultures are awaited.

PRINCIPLES OF TREATMENT

The mainstay of osteomyelitis treatment is prolonged, appropriate antibiotic therapy. The best results have been obtained with an initial course of 4–6 weeks of parenteral therapy followed by a similar period of oral treatment. Parenteral therapy gives reliable blood levels and promotes therapeutic bone and soft tissue levels of antibiotics. However, with newer antimicrobial agents, such as the quinolones, there is increasing interest in oral therapy for osteomyelitis. So far these approaches to therapy have not been subjected to adequate clinical trials.

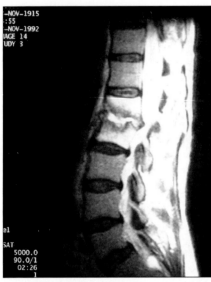

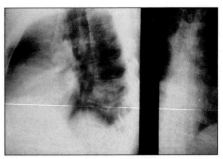

Fig. 12.10 *Plain X-ray showing vertebral osteomyelitis in brucellosis.*

Fig. 12.9 *MRI scan showing a high signal in acute staphylococcal lumbar discitis.*

In addition to antibiotics, surgery is usually required. Initially, surgery may be used to obtain diagnostic samples. However, it may also be required for debridement of infected soft tissue and bone and for excision of sequestra, the islands of dead bone that act as niduses for continued infection. Surgery is also required to remove infected prosthetic material.

Treatment progress should be monitored clinically and with suitable imaging. The role of inflammatory markers such as ESR and CRP in following disease progress is not established in osteomyelitis.

SPECIFIC ISSUES IN OSTEOMYELITIS

Vertebral osteomyelitis

Infection of the vertebrae is more common in adults than children and usually arises by the haematogenous route. The lower thoracic spine and the lumbar vertebrae are most frequently involved. There may be an initial discitis that spreads to the bone if not treated early enough (**Fig. 12.9**). Vertebral infection often presents with pain rather than systemic symptoms. Unchecked, complications include paravertebral abscesses and spinal cord compression. Although Gram-positive cocci such as staphylococci are often involved, there is an increasing incidence of disease due to Gram-negative bacilli, which may spread to the spine from the urinary tract either directly via the spinal venous plexus or following bacteraemia.

Plain X-rays are rarely helpful except in chronic osteomyelitis (**Fig. 12.10**). CT scans or MRI scans show inflammatory changes in the bones at a much earlier stage (**Fig. 12.11**).

An accurate bacteriological diagnosis should be made by bone biopsy, either done percutaneously or by an open procedure. Treatment requires prolonged antibiotics and often requires surgery, either to stabilize the spine if infection has caused vertebral collapse or to debride dead bone and paraspinal inflammatory tissue.

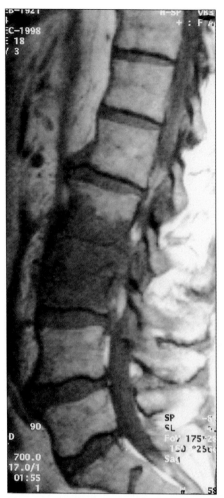

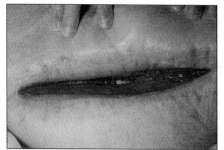

Fig. 12.12 *Infected hip prosthesis with wound breakdown to depth of prosthesis.*

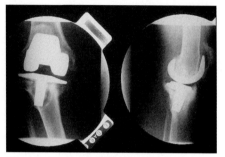

Fig. 12.13 *Loose tibial component in infected knee replacement.*

Fig. 12.11 *MRI scan showing bone and disc involvement in vertebral osteomyelitis.*

Prosthetic joints and other implanted devices

Joint replacements are now commonplace and some of these become infected (**Fig. 12.12**). Infection may occur at the time of implantation and present either acutely (in the immediate postoperative phase) or late. An artificial joint may also become infected if the patient becomes bacteraemic for some reason. Early infection is usually obvious, with wound breakdown and pus around the prosthesis. Late infection may present with new joint pain or with radiographic evidence of loosening of the prosthesis (**Fig. 12.13**).

In essence, there is osteomyelitis of the bone surrounding the prosthesis. If infection of a prosthetic joint is suspected, it is essential to obtain good specimens for microbiology either from joint aspiration or from formal exploration of the joint. Coagulase-negative staphylococci are the most common organisms found in this setting but some early infections are due to *S. aureus*, and this organism may also infect joints after an initial

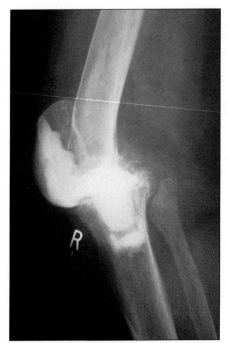

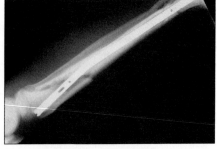

Fig. 12.15 *Infected tibial nail.*

Fig. 12.14 *Gentamicin-impregnated spacer following infected prosthetic knee excision.*

bacteraemia. Other skin commensals, such as *Propionobacterium* spp. and diphtheroids, may also cause prosthetic joint infection as, occasionally, may Gram-negative bacilli.

Management of these infections requires a combination of surgery and antibiotics. The joint needs to be revised either as a one-stage or a two-stage procedure. In a two-stage procedure the osteomyelitis is treated in the absence of the prosthetic joint and a new joint is implanted after the infection is cured. In the knee, a cement 'spacer' is required to preserve limb length (**Fig. 12.14**). Antibiotics need to be given parenterally for 4–6 weeks and sometimes for longer. Patients who are unfit for further surgery may be managed on oral antibiotics in an attempt to suppress the infection.

In addition to prosthetic joints, various metal devices are implanted into bone, usually to stabilize fractures or to correct deformity. These too may become infected with similar organisms to those that infect prostheses (**Fig. 12.15**); again *S. aureus* is the predominant pathogen. The resulting osteomyelitis is very difficult to eradicate until the metalwork is removed. Sometimes suppressive therapy must be given to contain the infection until the fracture has united and the metal can be removed, after which definitive therapy for the osteomyelitis can be given. External fixation devices may also be associated with infection (**Fig. 12.16**); these may be superficial pin-site infections or deeper infection involving the bone around a pin.

Diabetic feet

The combination of neuropathy and small vessel disease makes people with diabetes mellitus prone to soft tissue and bone infection in the lower limb, particularly in the foot. Osteomyelitis is likely if there is ulceration on the foot and, in particular, if a probe can reach bone when passed through the base of the ulcer (**Fig. 12.17**).

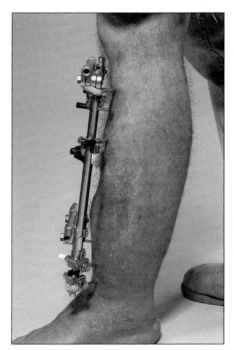

Fig. 12.16 *External fixation device for fractured tibia.*

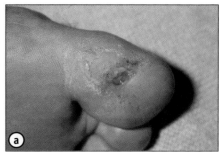

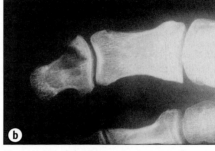

Fig. 12.17 *(a) Ulcer on great toe of diabetic; (b) Plain radiograph of same toe showing osteomyelitis in the terminal phalanx.*

If osteomyelitis is suspected, bone biopsy is required to obtain reliable microbiological specimens; swabs from ulcers are unreliable. Diabetic foot infections may be due to *S. aureus*, Gram-negative bacilli or anaerobes; often the infections are polymicrobial.

Treatment requires prolonged courses of antibiotics. Although conservative treatment is often attempted, debridement is frequently necessary and cure can sometimes be achieved only by amputation of the affected ray. Surgery is mandatory if there is severe or life-threatening sepsis.

Puncture wounds of the foot

A well-described cause of osteomyelitis of the bones of the feet is a puncture wound, usually with an iron nail that penetrates through the sole of a shoe, most commonly a 'trainer' or 'sneaker.' The infection is almost invariably due to *Pseudomonas aeruginosa*, possibly because these types of shoes tend to accumulate sweat that allows this micro-organism to colonize the inner lining of the shoe. This form of osteomyelitis can usually be readily treated with a prolonged course of an oral fluoroquinolone antibiotic.

Sickle cell disease

Patients with sickle cell disease are particularly prone to bone infection with *Salmonella* spp. Some series have also described infection with *S. aureus* and *Proteus mirabilis*. The fever and bone pain caused by osteomyelitis can be difficult to distinguish from a sickle crisis, so blood cultures should always be obtained. If fevers and rigors continue after a crisis, suspicion of osteomyelitis should be high.

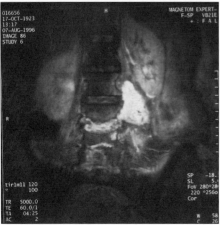

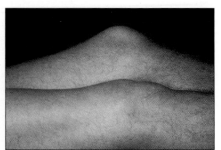

Fig. 12.19 *Acute streptococcal infection of the left knee.*

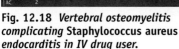

Fig. 12.18 *Vertebral osteomyelitis complicating* **Staphylococcus aureus** *endocarditis in IV drug user.*

Intravenous drug users

Injecting drug users are prone to bacteraemia and may, as a result, develop osteomyelitis (**Fig. 12.18**). The symptoms and signs may be subtle but, if suspected, bone biopsy is essential. *S. aureus*, Gram-negative bacilli (particularly *P. aeruginosa*) and *Candida* spp. are all possible pathogens in this setting.

SEPTIC ARTHRITIS

Joint infections may be caused by a variety of pathogens but bacteria are the most important. Organisms may enter the joint from adjacent tissues, may reach the joint via the bloodstream or may be introduced into the joint percutaneously. Patients with abnormal joints, such as those with rheumatoid disease or haemophilia, are more prone to develop septic arthritis.

The majority of adult cases of septic arthritis are due to *S. aureus*, with streptococci causing a significant minority. Gram-negative organisms may also cause septic arthritis, particularly in nosocomial infection. *Neisseria gonorrhoea* may present as a monoarthritis in disseminated gonococcal infection; this is often preceded by a polyarthralgia.

Septic arthritis usually presents with an acutely swollen and painful joint. The knee is the most commonly affected (**Fig. 12.19**), followed by the hip, ankle, wrist and shoulder. The affected joint is warm to the touch and there is usually clinical evidence of an effusion. The patient may be febrile but is rarely severely ill, and the peripheral leucocyte count may be normal in up to one-third of cases. In infection in abnormal joints, including prosthetic joints, the clinical signs may be subtle.

DIAGNOSIS

Diagnosis may be aided by plain X-rays or more sophisticated scanning, such as CT scan, but is most reliably made by aspiration of the affected joint. Gram stain reveals an organism in less than 70% of cases, so culture is essential. A leucocytosis in the joint fluid

(>50,000 leucocytes/ml) and a low glucose (<50% of the plasma glucose) are suggestive of infection, but similar findings may occur in an active rheumatoid joint. Many patients have positive blood cultures.

TREATMENT

Like other infections in closed spaces, successful treatment relies on correct antibiotic therapy and adequate joint drainage. Once an aspirate has been obtained for culture, empiric therapy should be started and should, at least, cover staphylococci and streptococci. The treatment should be widened if the patient is debilitated, immunocompromised or has a prosthetic joint. Parenteral therapy is usually given for at least 2 weeks, with a further 1–2 weeks of oral antibiotics. Children can sometimes be managed with oral therapy after an initial 48–72 hours of intravenous antibiotics.

In addition to antibiotics, some form of drainage procedure is mandatory. Repeated joint aspiration, arthroscopic washout or open surgical drainage can be used. Repeated needle aspiration is often successful in children but more formal drainage is required if the joint is not settling after 5 days. Adults require either a washout or open drainage. In very ill patients with multiple joint involvement following a bacteraemia, as may occur in rheumatoid disease, there is a place for repeated joint aspiration if the patient is too ill or frail for anaesthesia and joint surgery.

Patients also require analgesia, some form of rest splints and subsequent active physiotherapy.

Prosthetic joint infections rarely settle without removing the prosthesis. Reimplantation can occur once the infection has been cured with antibiotics.

VIRAL ARTHRITIS

A number of viral infections are associated with arthralgic or arthritis (**Fig 12.20**). Most cases of arthritis secondary to viral infections are relatively mild. Although virus can sometimes be recovered from joint fluid, many cases arise as a consequence of immunological phenomena affecting the synovium. There is usually a polyarthritis, but this is mild and does not last long. Only occasionally does joint damage occur.

REACTIVE ARTHRITIS

Some people get inflammatory arthritis following a bout of urethritis or dysentery (Reiter's syndrome) (see Chapter 10). This is highly associated with the HLA-B27 haplotype. Usually only one or two joints are involved, mainly in the lower limbs, and joint aspiration reveals scanty pus cells and no organisms. Molecular techniques have demonstrated chlamydial deoxyribonucleic acid in some cases of reactive arthritis associated with urethritis.

Viruses that may cause arthritis
Rubella
Hepatitis B
Adenovirus
Parvovirus
Mumps
Herpesviruses (Epstein–Barr virus, varicella-zoster virus)
Arthropod-borne alphaviruses (O'nyong-nyong fever virus, Chikungunya virus, Ross River virus)

Fig. 12.20 *Viruses that may cause arthritis.*

Treatment is with anti-inflammatory drugs and physiotherapy. Prolonged tetracycline therapy (for at least 3 months) may modify the disease in cases that are secondary to urethritis but not in those that follow dysentery. Many cases of reactive arthritis take many months to settle.

SEPTIC BURSITIS

The prepatellar bursa and the olecranon bursa are both prone to infection because the overlying skin is frequently subject to minor trauma. When infected, the bursa becomes inflamed and there is often some evidence of a portal of entry through the skin (**Fig. 12.21**). Fluid from the bursa can usually be aspirated and is purulent. The majority of cases are due to *S. aureus*. Needle drainage and parenteral antibiotics are sufficient in most cases but, occasionally, more formal drainage of the bursa is required.

TUBERCULOSIS

Although rare in developed countries, tuberculosis is still a common cause of bone and joint infection in the tropics. Most cases involve the spine. The knees and hips are the next most frequently infected but any joint may be involved. In the spine, infection starts in the anterior part of a vertebral body and invades through the disc to the adjacent vertebra. The resulting destruction may lead to an acute angulation of the spine, called a gibbus. The lower thoracic spine and the lumbar spine are the most commonly affected but the neck is sometimes involved. There may also be a paraspinal 'cold' abscess. Spinal cord compression is a not infrequent complication (**Fig. 12.22**). Other joints may present with pain, deformity or with a cold abscess (**Fig. 12.23**) and there may be a sinus (**Fig. 12.24**). The patient may have symptoms or signs of tuberculosis elsewhere.

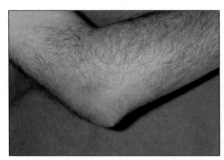

Fig. 12.21 *Acute olecranon bursitis caused by* Staphylococcus aureus.

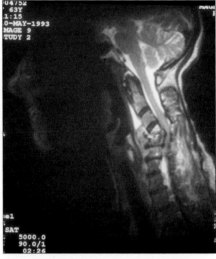

Fig. 12.22 *MRI scan showing gibbus in neck due to tuberculous osteomyelitis.*

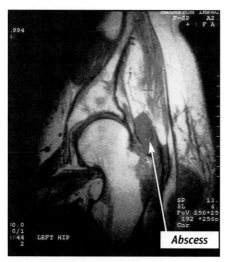

Abscess

Fig. 12.23 *MRI scan showing a 'cold abscess' around hip in tuberculosis.*

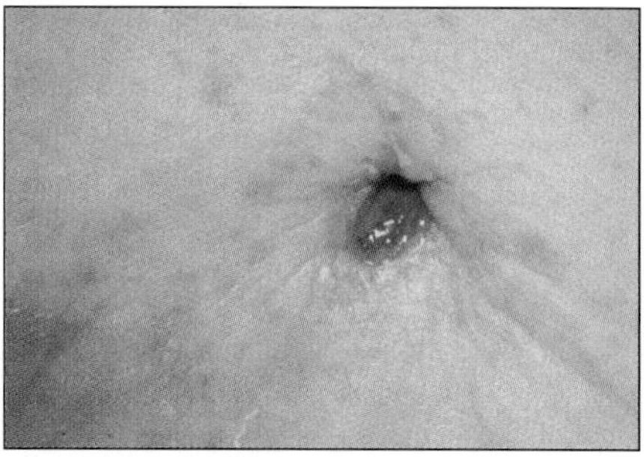

Fig. 12.24 *Sinus overlying the hip joint in tuberculosis of hip.*

DIAGNOSIS

Diagnosis depends on obtaining appropriate tissue for microscopy and culture. Joint fluid has a mixture of lymphocytes and neutrophils and it may have a low glucose level. There are visible acid-fast bacilli in the joint fluid in fewer than one-quarter of cases.

TREATMENT

The mainstay of treatment is antituberculous drug therapy with at least three agents for 6–9 months. Surgery is only required to treat cord compression or progressive deformity or to debride exuberant inflammatory tissue. However, even when surgery is not available, a surprising proportion of patients with neurological signs recover fully. Plaster jackets for spinal tuberculosis or limb immobilization for joint disease are not necessary.

chapter 13

The Immunocompromised Host

The immunocompromised host is one who has or develops a defect in the body's natural defense against microbial invasion. Such defects can arise from:

- local disruption of a host defense, such as the skin;
- systemic abnormalities of humoral or cellular immunity, such as congenital defects of T or B lymphocytes; or
- an acquired defect, such as exogenous immunosuppression owing to organ transplantation or infection with a virus such as the human immunodeficiency virus (HIV).

Figure 13.1 classifies the types of immunodeficiency and the organisms that most commonly occur as a complication of these various types of immunodeficiency.

Immune defects and commonly associated pathogens

Immune defect	Pathogens
Barrier breakdown	
Burns	*Pseudomonas aeruginosa, Staphylococcus aureus*
Trauma	*Streptococcus pyogenes, Staphylococcus epidermidis*
Phagocytic function	
Absolute decrease	Enteric Gram-negative bacteria, *Pseudomonas aeruginosa, Aspergillus* spp., *Candida* spp.
Chemotaxis	*Staphylococcus aureus*, enteric Gram-negative bacteria
Microbial killing	*Staphylococcus aureus, Burkholderia cepacia*, Gram-negative bacteria, *Aspergillus* spp.
Humoral immunity	
Hypogammaglobulinaemia	*Streptococcus pneumoniae, Haemophilus influenzae*
IgA deficiency	Pyogenic bacteria, *Giardia lamblia.*
Asplenia	*Streptococcus pneumoniae, Haemophilus influenzae*
Complement deficiency	Pyogenic bacteria, *Neisseria* spp.
Cell-mediated immunity	Intracellular bacteria (e.g. *Listeria* monocytogenes), viruses (e.g. Herpes family), fungi (e.g. *Candida* spp., *Cryptococcus* spp.), parasites (e.g. *Toxoplasma gondii*)

Fig. 13.1 *Immune defects and commonly associated pathogens. The list of pathogens is representative, but it is not intended to be all-inclusive.*

BARRIER DEFECTS

BURN WOUNDS

Burn wound injuries act as a direct insult to the mechanical protection afforded by skin. The burn wound surface serves as a nutritious physiological substrate for the growth of micro-organisms. Despite topical antimicrobial therapy the burn wound can become easily colonized. Pathogenic organisms such as *Staphylococcus aureus* and *Pseudomonas aeruginosa* can invade healthy tissue from the burn wound and then invade lymphatic vessels and cause direct blood stream invasion. Because of the moist environment in burn wounds *P. aeruginosa* is particularly problematic. The high rates of colonization of burn wound surfaces facilitates spread of organisms between patients, and outbreaks of infection with *P. aeruginosa* and methicillin-resistant *S. aureus* are common in burn units.

Therapy of burn wound infections typically requires broadly directed antimicrobial therapy and surgical debridement of nonviable tissues. Prevention of infection is a mainstay of the management of burn patients. Topical agents with antimicrobial activity, such as silver nitrate, are used to prevent colonization by micro-organisms. Maintenance of adequate disinfection and strict infection control policies may help to prevent the spread of infection.

TRAUMA

Trauma is another means by which micro-organisms traverse the integrity of the mechanical barrier of skin and cause infection. War wound injuries have historically lead to *Clostridium perfringens* infection (**Fig. 13.2**). Fortunately this is a rare occurrence today. When *C. perfringens* infection does occur as a result of traumatic injury, gross haemolysis of the red blood cells (**Fig. 13.3**) caused by α-toxin may occur.

Trauma may occur either accidentally or intentionally. Postoperative wound infections may occur, especially as a complication of surgery in a contaminated environment such as the colon. Mixed infections with aerobic and anaerobic microbial flora are the rule in such infections. Traumatic injury to an extremity, such as a cat bite or scratch may lead to an unusual organism, *Pasteurella multocida* (**Fig. 13.4**).

CATHETERS

The growth of the use of plastic catheters and artificial devices has placed patients in a compromised state by virtue of the foreign bodies that are present. Catheters of the urinary tract, intravenous access devices, peritoneal catheters for dialysis, prosthetic heart values,

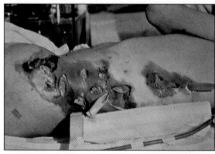

Fig. 13.2 *Gas gangrene due to* Clostridium perfringens.

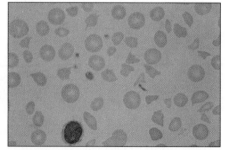

Fig. 13.3 *Haemolysis of red blood cells.*

Fig. 13.4 **Pasteurella multocida.**

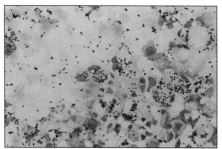

Fig. 13.5 *Gram stain of* **Staphylococcus epidermidis.**

and artificial joints all have a tendency to become infected with bacteria with low pathogenic potential, such as *Staphylococcus epidermidis* (**Fig. 13.5**) and *Propionibacterium acnes*, which tend to be commonly found on the skin and appear to have adherent properties.

Urinary catheters change normal urinary flow and disrupt the natural mechanical barrier. Furthermore, the catheter or drainage bag may become colonized through manipulation. In contrast to prosthetic devices, urinary catheters frequently become colonized with fecal flora. Gram-negative organisms, enterococci and *Candida* spp. become important pathogens in the setting of prolonged urinary catheterization.

NORMAL FLORA

Normal bacterial flora may be disrupted in the gastrointestinal tract, typically through the use of antimicrobial agents. The decrease in normal flora results in a change in microenvironment of the gut and may predispose patients to such problems as antibiotic-associated colitis due to *Clostridium difficile*.

Another barrier that is occasionally abrogated is the lungs, where mucus production, ciliary clearance from respiratory epithelial cells and an effective cough reflex serve to trap micro-organisms and prevent passage into the lungs. The most extreme example of this problem is patients with cystic fibrosis, a disease of genetic origin in which abnormally thick mucus is produced (**Fig. 13.6**), coupled with a number of metabolic abnormalities. The most common organisms causing pneumonia in this condition are *P. aeruginosa* (**Fig. 13.7**) and *Burkholderia cepacia*. *B. cepacia* has recently been recognized as a pathogen in patients with cystic fibrosis and requires specific media for isolation (**Fig. 13.8**).

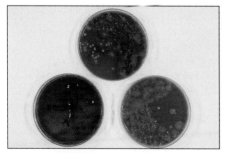

Fig. 13.6 *Sputum from a patient with cystic fibrosis.*

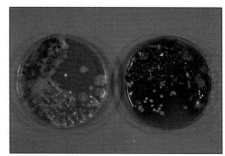

Fig. 13.7 *Colonies of* **Pseudomonas aeruginosa** *from the sputum of a patient with cystic fibrosis.*

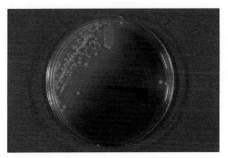

Fig. 13.8 Burkholderia cepacia *on a plate (selective media).*

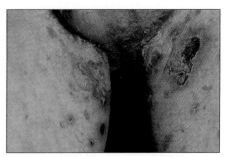

Fig. 13.9 *Skin lesion of ecthyma gangrenosum.*

ABNORMALITIES OF HUMORAL OR CELLULAR IMMUNITY

ABNORMALITIES OF PHAGOCYTIC FUNCTION

The presence of neutrophils serves a critical function in checking the spread of infection. Defects in neutrophil quantity predispose patients to bacterial infection; there is a predictable relationship between the likelihood of infection and the absolute granulocyte count. Neutropenia (defined as less than 0.5×10^6 neutrophils/ml) is associated with a marked increase in the rate of infection and bacteraemia. The organisms typically associated with neutropenia are the patient's own flora, frequently enteric Gram-negative bacilli, *P. aeruginosa* and *Candida* spp. As granulocytopenia persists the risk of infection with *Candida* spp. and *Aspergillus* spp. increases.

The presentation of neutropenia and fever is frequently nonspecific, without an obvious focus of infection. Occasionally bacteraemic spread of organisms such as *P. aeruginosa* leads to ecthyma gangrenosum (**Fig. 13.9**), a necrotic ulceration of the skin. Although this is typically due to *Pseudomonas aeruginosa*, ecthyma can be caused by other Gram-negative organisms and even by *S. aureus*.

Because of the potentially rapid demise of patients with fever and neutropenia, antimicrobial therapy must be started rapidly and directed broadly at all potential pathogens until results of culture are available. Use of myelopoietic-stimulating factors such as granulocyte colony stimulating factor may shorten the period of fever and neutropenia and hasten recovery.

Chemotactic abnormalities of phagocytes are rare and usually congenital. There are a number of well-characterized chemotactic defects, including abnormal attraction to chemoattractants, poor or absent locomotion, and poor signaling. Patients with congenital neutrophil disorders are usually afflicted with recurrent *S. aureus* infections.

An interesting and well-characterized physiologic defect of polymorphonuclear microbial killing power is chronic granulomatous disease (CGD). This is a disease in which neutrophils fail to mount a respiratory burst during phagocytosis due to a deficiency in the enzyme NADPH oxidase. The consequence of this defect is a lack of formation of hydrogen peroxide. Patients with CGD are at risk from infections with:

- catalase-positive organisms such as *S. aureus* (**Fig. 13.10**);
- Gram-negative organisms such as *Serratia marcescens* or *B. cepacia*; and
- *Aspergillus* spp.

In contrast, organisms such as the pneumococcus or other streptococci make their own hydrogen peroxide and can be killed by the neutrophils of CGD patients because they

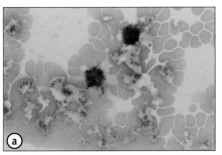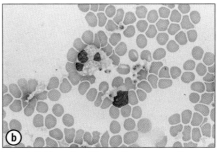

Fig. 13.10 *Chronic granulomatous disease (CGD): (a) The nitroblue toluene test shows the ingestion of the dye by normal neutrophils in the control patient but no uptake by polymorphs from a patient with CGD(b).*

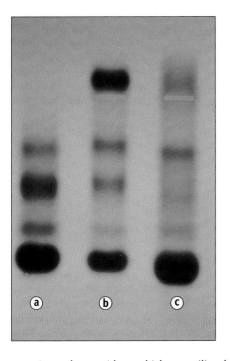

Fig. 13.11 *Serum protein electrophoresis: (a) hypogammaglobulinaemia; (b) paraprotein band; (c) normal.*

contain myeloperoxidase, which can utilize the bacteria's own hydrogen peroxide to cause killing. There is some evidence that CGD patients can be successfully treated with γ-interferon, which restores some of the defect. Prophylactic antibiotics may also be useful.

ABNORMALITIES OF HUMORAL IMMUNITY

Immunoglobulin deficiency typically results in recurrent upper or lower respiratory tract disease caused by encapsulated bacteria, underscoring the importance of antibody in the opsonization of such bacteria. Immunoglobulin deficiency can be congenital (Bruton's X-linked agammaglobulinemia) or acquired (such as in common variable immunodeficiency) (Fig. 13.11). Transient hypogammaglobulinemia of infancy is a condition that is characterized by recurrent respiratory infections, associated with low immunoglobulin (Ig) G levels; it may normalize by the age of 4 years. There are also

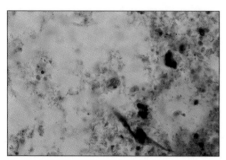

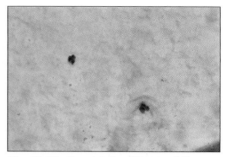

Fig. 13.12 *Trophozoite of* Giardia lamblia.   Fig. 13.13 *Gram stain of* Haemophilus influenzae.

immunoglobulin subclass deficiencies such as absent IgG_2 or IgG_4, which may lead to recurrent infections, similar to those seen with complete absence of gammaglobulin. Deficiency of IgA, which may occur in certain conditions such as ataxia telangiectasia, may lead to intestinal infection with the parasite *Giardia lamblia* (**Fig. 13.12**).

There are a number of other conditions that can lead to functional or quantitative defects in immunoglobulin, such as multiple myeloma or conditions that lead to protein loss (e.g. nephrotic syndrome). Regardless of the cause of immunoglobulin dysfunction, one of the hallmarks of infection is recurrent infection from encapsulated bacteria such as *Streptococcus pneumoniae* or *Haemophilus influenzae* (**Fig. 13.13**).

The mainstay of therapy of immunoglobulin deficiency is immunoglobulin replacement therapy whereby monthly intravenous infusions of IgG are given to reduce the rate of infection.

ABNORMALITIES OF COMPLEMENT

The complement system is a series of proteins that promote defence against microbes by:
- enhancing susceptibility to phagocytosis;
- lysing some bacteria directly
- producing chemotactic factors for polymorphonuclear leucocytes; and
- promoting the inflammatory response.

Complement deficiency is rare and when it occurs leads to a predisposition to infection with encapsulated bacteria. *Neisseria* spp., in particular *Neisseria meningitidis*, are a special problem for patients who have defects in the terminal portion of the complement cascade. Patients with such a deficiency may present with recurrent meningococcaemia (**Fig. 13.14**). Most clinically significant defects of the complement system are congenital in origin.

DEFECTS IN CELLULAR IMMUNITY

Defects in cellular immunity may be classified as either congenital or acquired. The most common acquired defects seen today are those caused by infection with HIV type 1 and those brought about by exogenous immunosuppression to preserve a transplanted organ. Both are discussed in some detail below.

Congenital anomalies of cellular function may affect both T and B lymphocytes. When both occur, the outcome, severe combined immunodeficiency, is incompatible with life. However, defects limited to T lymphocytes (e.g. Di George syndrome) are compatible with life. Such patients have recurrent infection due to a variety of pathogens that survive intracellularly; these include as cytomegalovirus (CMV), *Pneumocystis carinii*, *Candida* spp. and mycobacteria.

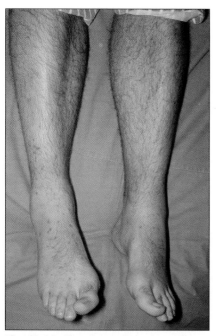

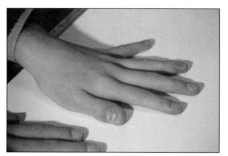

Fig. 13.15 *Chronic mucocutaneous candidiasis.*

Fig. 13.14 *Chronic meningococcaemia rash.*

Chronic mucocutaneous candidiasis (**Fig. 13.15**) is one consequence of either congenital or acquired defects in T-lymphocyte function. Chronic mucocutaneous candidiasis is characterized by persistent but noninvasive infection of mucous membranes, hair, skin or nails in patients who have a specific defect in T-lymphocyte function that renders them anergic to *Candida* spp. Treatment may require chronic suppressive doses of antifungal agents such as ketoconazole, miconazole or fluconazole.

ORGAN TRANSPLANTATION

Organ transplant recipients are typically affected by a variety of pathogens that tend to survive intracellularly, since the immunosuppressive medications that are used to preserve the graft are directed at the cellular immune system. Although always at risk for the typical postoperative complications, such as pneumonia, wound or urinary tract infection, these patients tend to go through a predictable time interval during which the risk of certain pathogens predominates (**Fig. 13.16**).

VIRAL INFECTIONS

Two viral infections predominate in the early postoperative periods: herpes simplex virus (HSV), which usually manifests as recurrence of mucocutaneous disease, and CMV. Recurrent HSV infection is generally either prevented or treated in the early post-transplant period with aciclovir.

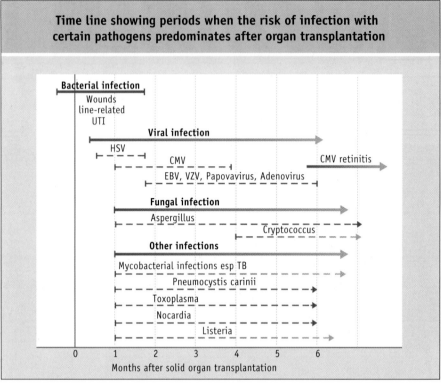

Time line showing periods when the risk of infection with certain pathogens predominates after organ transplantation

Fig. 13.16 *Time line showing periods when the risk of infection with certain pathogens predominates after organ transplantation.*

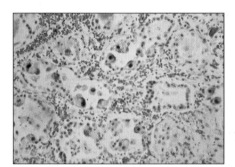

Fig. 13.17 *Lung biopsy showing cytomegalovirus inclusions.*

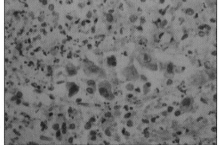

Fig. 13.18 *Lung biopsy of cytomegalovirus pneumonia in a transplant recipient (magnified view).*

Cytomegalovirus is the most significant pathogen to complicate organ transplantation. The virus has direct effects on the host by causing fever, leukopenia, hepatitis and occasionally pneumonia (**Figs 13.17** and **13.18**). The virus is also thought to predispose to concomitant infection with other pathogens that live intracellularly, such as *Nocardia* spp.,

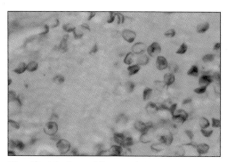

Fig. 13.19 *Lung biopsy of* Pneumocystis carinii *and cytomegalovirus pneumonia.*

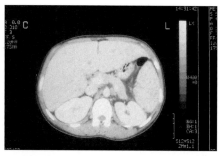

Fig. 13.20 *Disseminated candidiasis in a transplant recipient.*

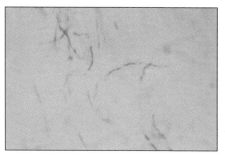

Fig. 13.21 *Gram stain of* Nocardia *organisms.*

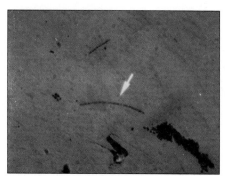

Fig. 13.22 *Modified acid-fast stain of* Nocardia *organisms.*

P. carinii (**Fig. 13.19**) and *Candida* spp. (**Fig. 13.20**). *Nocardia* spp. have a worldwide distribution. The lung is generally the most common site of infection, but central nervous system or skin involvement is not uncommon. *Nocardia* spp. are slow growing and the laboratory must be alerted so that it can make proper attempts at isolation and avoid overgrowth from other flora. The organisms are Gram-negative or Gram-variable (**Fig. 13.21**) branching rods that are weakly acid fast (**Fig. 13.22**).

In addition, CMV appears to contribute to graft dysfunction and may be associated with decreased long-term survival. The peak time for occurrence of CMV disease is 4–12 weeks post-transplant. The source of the infection is generally latent virus from the transplanted organ. However, if the patient has previously been infected with CMV then the course of immunosuppression may lead to reactivation of latent infection.

Diagnosis of CMV disease rests on histological confirmation of the virus in tissue (**Fig. 13.23**). Because the virus may take weeks to grow in tissue culture, more rapid methods are being used to detect the virus, such as centrifugation-enhanced (shell vial) culture with monoclonal antibody staining (**Fig. 13.24**), the polymerase chain reaction or direct staining of blood leucocytes for CMV antigens. Therapy or prevention with an effective antiviral agent such as ganciclovir, with or without the use of CMV-specific hyperimmunoglobulin, is the current standard of management.

Other viral infections, most notably with hepatitis B virus and hepatitis C virus, may also complicate organ transplantation, especially liver transplantation.

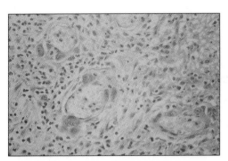

Fig. 13.23 *Cytomegalovirus in the colon showing typical intracellular inclusions.*

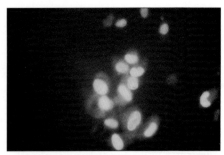

Fig. 13.24 *Positive cytomegalovirus shell vial stain in culture.*

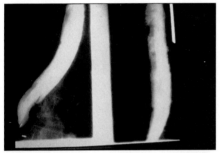

Fig. 13.25 *Barium swallow in oesophageal candidiasis.*

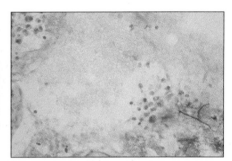

Fig. 13.26 *Candidal osteomyelitis.*

FUNGAL INFECTIONS

There are a number of fungal infections that complicate organ transplantation. In the early postoperative period, *Candida* spp., as nosocomial pathogens, often predominate. Oropharyngeal candidiasis may cause sore throat and difficulty in swallowing (**Fig. 13.25**). In a significant proportion of transplant patients disseminated candidal infection may lead to abscesses in the liver, osteomyelitis of spine (**Fig. 13.26**) or sepsis.

As a later manifestation of immunosuppression, exposure to more inherently pathogenic fungi such as *Cryptococcus* spp., *Histoplasma* spp. and *Coccidioides* spp. may occur; the particular fungi involved depend on the geographical region where the patient lives.

Cryptococcal infection in transplant recipients presents as fever, with or without headache and signs of meningitis. Onset of disease may be slow, and occasionally sites such as bone, joints or skin may be involved. It can occur at any time after discharge from hospital but typically occurs within the first year post-transplant. It is more frequent in patients who have higher levels of immunosuppression because of chronic rejection. Patients have organisms detectable in the cerebrospinal fluid (CSF); the organisms are characterized by their large capsule, which can be seen on India ink preparation (**Fig. 13.27**) or by using a latex agglutination assay to detect the presence of antigen (**Fig. 13.28**). Therapy with antifungal agents such as amphotericin B or fluconazole is usually successful if the infection is detected before the onset of significant neurological deficit. In transplant recipients, monitoring of CSF or serum titres of cryptococcal antigen may be useful as a guide to successful therapy.

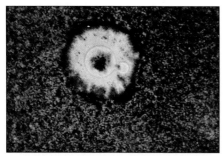

Fig. 13.27 *India ink preparation showing cryptococcal capsule and budding yeast.*

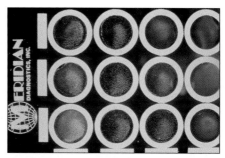

Fig. 13.28 *Latex agglutination showing cryptococcal antigen.*

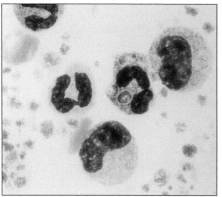

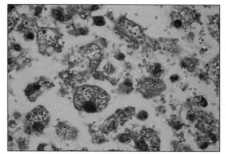

Fig. 13.30 *Tissue histology of Histoplasma capsulatum.*

Fig. 13.29 *Buffy coat smear showing* **Histoplasma capsulatum** *within the cytoplasm of a neutrophil (Giemsa stain).*

Histoplasma capsulatum is a pathogenic fungus that typically infects many normal people living in endemic areas; however, it tends to cause progressive disseminated disease in immunosuppressed patients. In normal hosts, the organism presents as a benign self-limited pulmonary infection. The natural habitat is the soil; it is found in the central region of the USA surrounding the plane of the Mississippi River and in some areas of the Caribbean, such as Haiti and Puerto Rico. Disseminated disease may occur years after initial infection upon the development of significant immunosuppression. Cultures of blood, bone marrow, sputum, CSF or urine have yielded the organism (**Fig. 13.29**). Often biopsy or histological examination of tissue may be required to make the diagnosis (**Fig. 13.30**). A serum or urinary antigen test is available and this may also be used to make a diagnosis; it can additionally be used to monitor effectiveness of therapy. Amphotericin B is generally required for therapy.

Coccidioides immitis is found in the south-western USA. As with histoplasmosis, infection with this fungus generally affects large numbers of people living in the endemic area. Usually the presentation is pulmonary in origin; however, dissemination is common in immunosuppressed patients. Sites of dissemination include the meninges, bones and skin. Infection can be documented by biopsy of affected material (**Fig. 13.31**). Therapy of coccidioidomycosis requires antifungal therapy with amphotericin B, sometimes intrathecally, for prolonged periods of time.

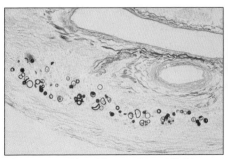

Fig. 13.31 *Tissue biopsy of* Coccidioides immitis.

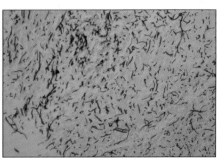

Fig. 13.32 *Oesophageal candidiasis.*

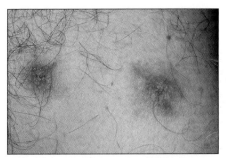

Fig. 13.33 *Disseminated candidiasis.*

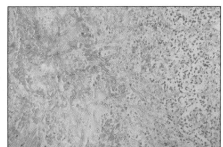

Fig. 13.34 *Aspergillosis in lungs of a bone marrow transplant recipient.*

BONE MARROW TRANSPLANTATION

Infections in patients with haematological malignancy occur because of lack of circulating neutrophils from marrow failure. Neutropenia may persist for days or weeks after either intensive chemotherapy or marrow transplantation. The duration of neutropenia influences the type of infectious problem. In the early phase of neutropenia, patients are subject to Gram-negative bacteraemia. Such patients are at risk of infections such as ecthyma gangrenosum (see **Fig. 13.9**) which are classifically caused by *P. aeruginosa*. In prolonged neutropenia, fungal infections such as candidiasis and aspergillosis become more common.

Among bone marrow transplant recipients, disseminated candidiasis can occur by spread through the intestinal wall from the gastrointestinal tract (**Figs 13.32** and **13.33**). Diagnosis may be difficult and it requires a strong index of suspicion. Fever that is persistent despite adequate antimicrobial therapy directed at bacterial pathogens in neutropenic patients may prompt empiric antifungal therapy. Blood cultures may turn positive in about half the cases of dissemination.

Aspergillosis is a potentially lethal complication among immunocompromised patients. Although *Aspergillus* spp. are not as invasive as *Histoplasma* spp. or *Coccidioidomycoses* spp., these organisms are ubiquitous and are typically found in soil, dust and moist environments. Bone marrow transplantation patients are particularly vulnerable. Infection starts via inhalation and spreads to the sinuses or lungs (**Fig. 13.34**). Dissemination to the central nervous system (**Fig. 13.35**), the heart (**Fig. 13.36**) or local invasion from sinus

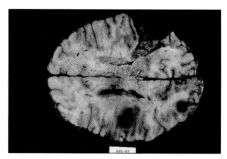

Fig. 13.35 Aspergillus *brain abscess.*

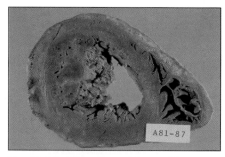

Fig. 13.36 *Disseminated* Aspergillus *involving the heart.*

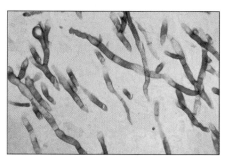

Fig. 13.37 *Stain of* Aspergillus *in lung.*

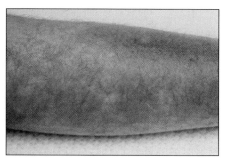

Fig. 13.38 *Skin rash in graft-versus-host disease.*

infection may lead to abscess formation. Invasive aspergillosis (**Fig. 13.37**) has a very high fatality rate because of the difficulty of diagnosis, the relative insensitivity of the organisms to antifungal agents and their pathogenic potential.

Aggressive antifungal therapy and reconstitution of immunity with granulocyte colony stimulating factors may help to improve survival. Because of the ubiquity of the organism and the predictability of risk in marrow transplantation patients (as well as other immunocompromised patients), hospitals have taken steps to protect patients by using high efficiency particulate filters for air handling in selected rooms where these patients are housed.

Among bone marrow transplant recipients, CMV interstitial pneumonitis is also a potentially lethal complication. In contrast to the situation in solid organ transplantation, CMV pneumonia in this population is poorly responsive to therapy with antiviral agents alone. In fact, the process is thought to be more akin to an immunopathological event, requiring combination antiviral and immunoglobulin therapy.

Another factor associated with the development of infectious complications in bone marrow transplantation is the development of graft-versus-host disease. Such development may occur in association with CMV, and is a predisposing factor in patients who develop CMV disease. Graft-versus-host disease may present with fever, diarrhoea, skin rash (**Fig. 13.38**) and abnormalities of liver function; all of these presentations can mimic an infectious process. The therapy for graft-versus-host disease, which is increased immunosuppression, may increase the risk of infectious complications.

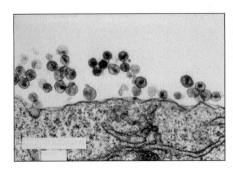

Fig. 13.39 *Electron micrograph showing replicating HIV: new virus particles budding from the surface of a lymphocyte in tissue culture.*

HUMAN IMMUNODEFICIENCY VIRUS

By far the most common form of immunosuppression seen in the world today is infection due to HIV type 1. Acquired immunodeficiency syndrome (AIDS), caused by infection with HIV type 1, was first recognized in 1980 as a syndrome and was first defined by the isolation of HIV type 1 in 1984. There are now about 3 million cases of AIDS and approximately 15 million HIV-infected people worldwide.

The virus, HIV type 1, infects T lymphocytes (CD4+ cells) as well as other tissues and cells throughout the body, including plasma cells, macrophages, brain and semen. With bursts of viral replication (**Fig. 13.39**) there is an inexorable decline in CD4+ (helper) T lymphocytes, which leads to decreased cellular immunity. There is a very strong and direct association between the risk of opportunistic infection with intracellular pathogens and the level of the CD4+ T-lymphocyte count (**Fig. 13.40**).

HIV type 1 is a member of the retrovirus family. These viruses are small lipid-enveloped ribonucleic acid viruses that contain reverse transcriptase. There are three important genes:
- one gene (*env*) codes for envelope glycoproteins;
- one gene (*pol*) codes the polymerase genes for reverse transcriptase; and
- one gene (*gag*) codes for a number of core proteins.

Once infected, the patient harbours virus in a latent state; however, widespread replication and viral turnover occur daily with destruction of CD4+ T lymphocyte lines.

Among the unique responses to HIV infection is the inability of the host to halt viral replication. The tests used to diagnose HIV infection rely on the major structural proteins of this retrovirus. Once a patient is infected, it may take weeks or months to develop detectable antibody to HIV (**Fig. 13.41**). Seroconversion can be detected by the presence of serum antibody to HIV on enzyme immunoassay followed by confirmation testing using Western blotting techniques (**Fig. 13.42**). There are criteria for classification of a positive Western blot – most authorities require the presence of at least two of the following bands: p24 or p31; gp41; or gp 120/160.

Recent attention has focused on 'viral load' measurements using molecular techniques for the monitoring and treatment of HIV infection; HIV ribonucleic acid viral load has been shown to be directly correlated to progression of disease and effectiveness of antiretroviral therapy (**Fig. 13.43**).

HIV is transmitted by:
- sexual contact (both homosexual and heterosexual);
- injection drug use;
- mother-to-infant transmission; and
- transfusion with contaminated blood and blood factor concentrates.

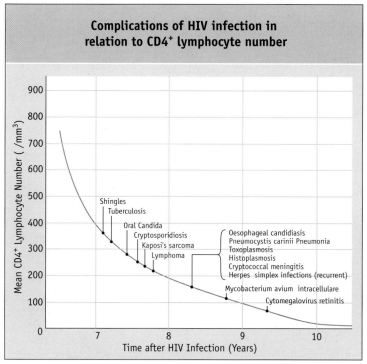

Complications of HIV infection in relation to CD4⁺ lymphocyte number

Fig. 13.40 *Decline of CD4⁺ lymphocytes over time in HIV infection.*

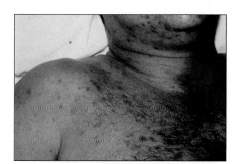

Fig. 13.41 *Seroconversion rash in HIV type 1 infection.*

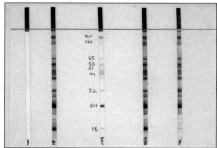

Fig. 13.42 *Western blot of serum from a person with HIV infection.*

The risk to health care workers following needle-stick injury is very small, approximately 3 per 1000 such injuries.

There appear to be effective means of preventing transmission of HIV infection through the use of:

- barrier precautions during sexual contact;
- precautions when handling blood and contaminated bodily fluids;
- screening of donors contributing to the blood supply
- the use of artificial or pasteurized clotting factor concentrates; and
- the treatment of HIV carrier mothers and their newborn babies with antiretroviral therapy.

203

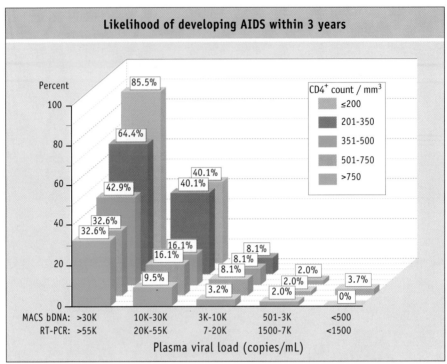

Fig. 13.43 *Viral load in relation to disease progression in HIV type 1 infection.*

Initial (primary) HIV infection may manifest as a 'mononucleosis-like' illness characterized by fever, lymphadenopathy, sore throat, malaise and fatigue. Occasionally, patients have an aseptic meningitis and, more rarely, other neurological manifestations such as myelopathy, radiculopathy or Guillain–Barré syndrome. When it occurs, primary illness is usually seen 2–4 weeks following onset of infection.

The inexorable decline in CD4+ (helper) T lymphocytes leads to a marked degree of susceptibility to a number of pathogens that are primarily intracellular (**Fig. 13.44**). In contrast to organ or bone marrow transplantation patients, HIV-infected patients can have no reconstitution of immune function or reduction in their levels of immunosuppression. Therefore, many of the infections that occur are very likely to persist, progress or relapse unless effective therapy or prophylaxis is maintained. Infections that are relatively self-limiting for the average patient, such as salmonellosis, have a tendency to relapse without long-term therapy. Cytomegalovirus retinitis requires life-long prevention, as does cryptococcal infection. (In contrast, transplant patients frequently recover after effective therapy for these pathogens and recurrence is uncommon.) The use of highly active antiretroviral therapy (HAART) has led to a sharp decline in the incidence of opportunist infections in people with HIV.

PNEUMOCYSTIS CARINII INFECTION

The most common infection among HIV-positive patients is *P. carinii* pneumonia. *P. carinii* has been an organism of uncertain classification; it was previously classified as a parasite, more recently it has been classified as a fungus. The organism is ubiquitous. Antibody

Pathogens in HIV infection

	Infecting organism	Type of infection
Viruses	Cytomegalovirus	Pneumonia, disseminated infection, retinitis, encephalitis
	Epstein–Barr virus	Important pathogenic factor in B-cell lymphoproliferative disorders and Burkitt's lymphoma, oral hairy leukoplakia
	Herpes simplex virus	Recurrent severe localized infection
	Varicella-zoster virus	Localized or disseminated infection
	Papovavirus	Progressive multifocal leukoencephalopathy
Fungi	*Candida albicans*	Mucocutaneous infection, esophagitis, disseminated infection
	Cryptococcus neoformans	Meningitis, disseminated infection
	Histoplasma capsulatum	Disseminated infection
	Coccidioides immitis	Disseminated infection
	Petriellidium boydii	Pneumonia
	Aspergillus spp.	Invasive pulmonary infection with potential for dissemination
Protozoa	*Pneumocystis carinii*	Pneumonia, retinal infection
	Toxoplasma gondii	Encephalitis
	Cryptosporidium parvum	Enteritis
	Isospora belli	Enteritis
	Microsporidia	Enteritis
Mycobacteria	*Mycobacterium avium*	Disseminated infection complex
	Mycobacterium tuberculosis	Disseminated infection, pneumonia
Bacteria	*Nocardia* spp.	Pneumonia, disseminated infection
	Legionella spp.	Pneumonia
	Streptococcus pneumoniae	Pneumonia, disseminated infection
	Haemophilus influenzae type B	Pneumonia, disseminated infection
	Salmonella spp.	Gastroenteritis, disseminated infection

Fig. 13.44 *Pathogens in HIV infection.*

testing has demonstrated widespread distribution in the population. It has been presumed that the vast majority of cases in HIV-infected patients are due to reactivation. The primary presentation is fever, cough and shortness of breath. Clinical examination of the chest is usually normal, but the chest radiograph typically shows bilateral perihilar infiltrates (**Fig. 13.45**). The lungs are the site in the body where the organism manifests itself. Diagnosis can be made by silver stain of induced sputum, bronchoalveolar lavage or lung biopsy (**Fig. 13.46**). Treatment with co-trimoxazole with or without corticosteroids is often successful. After they have been treated, patients infected with HIV require lifelong prophylaxis against *P. carinii* pneumonia because of the high likelihood of relapse.

CYTOMEGALOVIRUS INFECTION

Cytomegalovirus plays an important role in HIV-infected patients, as it does in transplant recipients. The primary clinical manifestation in the HIV-infected population is retinitis,

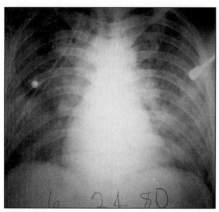

Fig. 13.45 *Chest X-ray of* **Pneumocystis carinii** *in HIV infection.*

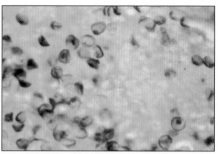

Fig. 13.46 *Lung biopsy in* **Pneumocystis carinii** *infection.*

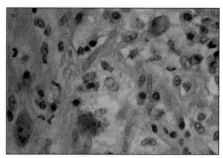

Fig. 13.47 *Cytomegalovirus appendicitis in a patient infected with HIV.*

although gastrointestinal involvement (even mimicking acute appendicitis) (**Fig. 13.47**), pulmonary involvement, central nervous system involvement or disseminated infection can occur. Cytomegalovirus meningoencephalitis can be particularly difficult to treat (**Fig. 13.48**). Therapy with antiviral agents directed at CMV are used to control the retinitis in order to prevent blindness. The patient requires life-long prophylaxis unless effective antiretroviral therapy can increase cell-mediated immunity.

MYCOBACTERIAL INFECTIONS

Mycobacterial infections in HIV infection are very common. Unique among these organisms is the tendency of *Mycobacterium tuberculosis* to disseminate. There is a very high incidence of disseminated *M. tuberculosis* among HIV-infected patients living in tropical and developing countries. In addition, atypical mycobacteria, such as *Mycobacterium avium-intercellulare* complex, are very common in such severely immunosuppressed patients. These organisms are generally not pathogenic for nonimmunosuppressed patients and are part of a group of the atypical mycobacteria that infect HIV-infected patients. Antituberculous drug resistance is the rule with *M. avium-intercellulare* complex, although newly developed agents such as the quinolones, clarithromycin, azithromycin and rifabutin have some activity against them.

Both *M. tuberculosis* and *M. avium-intercellulare* complex can be isolated from a variety of tissues and from blood, sputum or stool. In fact mycobacteraemia is not an uncommon event. Rapid and improved culture methods have improved our diagnostic ability, including isolation of mycobacteria from blood. Genetic probes can be used to make a molecular

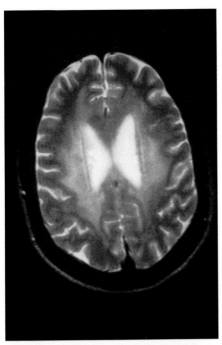

Fig. 13.49 *Liver biopsy of tuberculosis without granulomas in a patient infected with HIV.*

Fig. 13.48 *MRI scan of cytomegalovirus meningoencephalitis in a patient infected with HIV.*

diagnosis. One of the pathological features in many patients infected with both HIV and tuberculosis is the absence of classic necrotizing granuloma on tissue histology (**Fig. 13.49**).

PARASITIC INFECTIONS
Toxoplasmosis
There are a number of parasitic infections that occur in HIV-infected patients. The most common of these is toxoplasmosis, which most frequently presents in HIV infection as a cause of seizures with a mass-forming lesion in the central nervous system. Computed tomography or magnetic resonance imaging scans (**Fig. 13.50**) frequently show multiple lesions, which on biopsy reveal the characteristic cysts of *Toxoplasma gondii* (**Fig. 13.51**).

Diagnosis can also be made through the use of diagnostic serologic assays for IgM antibody or with molecular probes of affected tissue. Often presumptive therapy is undertaken of an HIV-infected patient with a central nervous system lesion and evidence of past exposure (by serology for IgG antibody) to *T. gondii*.

The treatment of choice is a combination of pyrimethamine and sulfadiazine. Alternative therapies include trimethoprim-sulphamethoxazole or a combination of clindamycin and primaquine. The use of co-trimoxazole for prophylaxis of *P. carinii* pneumonia has reduced dramatically the rate of reactivation of toxoplasmosis.

Cryptosporidiosis
Cryptosporidia are parasites of the intestine that have only been recently recognized as causing disease in humans. The development of disease, manifested by diffuse watery diarrhoea, was first recognized in HIV-infected patients. Although outbreaks have occurred

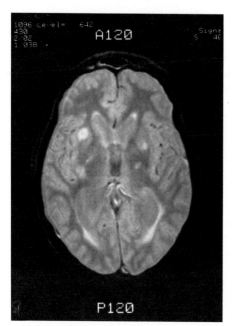

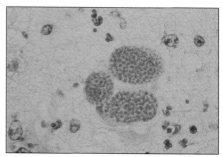

Fig. 13.51 *Cysts of* Toxoplasma gondii *in a brain biopsy.*

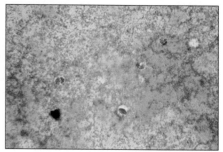

Fig. 13.50 *MRI showing toxoplasmosis of the central nervous system.*

Fig. 13.52 *Cryptosporidia in stool.*

in relation to contaminated water supplies in a few unusual outbreaks, the majority of cases are sporadic. In a normal host, the diarrhoea is generally self-limiting; however, in HIV-infected patients, the diarrhoea may be very profuse, even 'cholera-like', and unrelenting. Diagnosis can be made by performing a modified acid-fast stain of the stool (**Fig. 13.52**).

Effective specific therapy directed toward cryptosporidial infection in HIV-infected patients is not available. Many patients have profound and life-threatening weight loss.

Other parasitic infections

Another parasite of limited importance in the nonimmunosuppressed host but of some clinical significance in HIV-infected patients is *Isospora belli* (**Fig. 13.53**). It may produce severe diarrhoea in AIDS patients. Unlike cryptosporidia, it is responsive to antimicrobial therapy with trimethoprim-sulfamethoxazole.

Other recently described protozoan parasites that may cause intestinal illness are microsporidia. There are a number of species, but *Enterocytozoon bieneusi* is the most common. Although gastroenteritis (**Fig. 13.54**) is the most frequent manifestation, a number of species have been known to involve the respiratory tract and eyes and to disseminate to muscles. Cytology of affected fluid or stool examination with a special stain may establish the diagnosis, although the small size of the organisms makes this difficult. Electron microscopy of affected tissues or small bowel biopsy with light microscopy may confirm the diagnosis.

LATENT VIRUSES

HIV also enhances the replication of other viruses of latency. Cytomegalovirus is but one example that has already been discussed. HSV in the HIV-infected patient is characterized

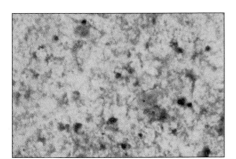

Fig. 13.53 **Isospora belli** *in stool.*

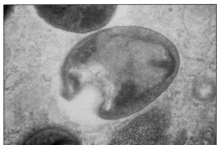

Fig. 13.54 *Electron micrograph of* Enterocytozoon bieneusi *in the stool from a patient with microsporidiosis complicating HIV infection.*

Fig. 13.55 *Perianal lesion of HSV in a patient infected with HIV.*

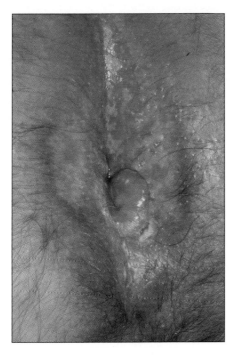

by very large, aggressive and progressive ulcerative lesions (**Fig. 13.55**). These lesions are frequently difficult to treat and may relapse after cessation of therapy. Patients with HIV infection are at risk of recurrence of herpes zoster (as are all immunosuppressed patients). Dissemination may occur (**Fig. 13.56**). Patients require aggressive antiviral therapy.

The polyomaviruses are small, nonenveloped deoxyribonucleic acid viruses that are widespread in the population. The JC and BK viruses from this family have been associated with progressive multifocal encephalopathy. The family of polyomaviruses are antigenically related to the monkey SV40 virus and other animal viruses. Asymptomatic excretion can occur with immunosuppression. Infection is very common.

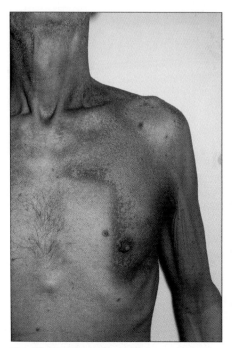

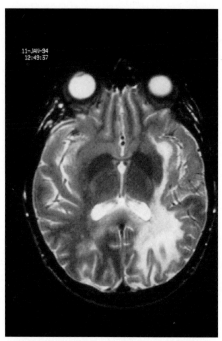

Fig. 13.56 *Disseminated herpes zoster in a man with HIV following radiotherapy for localized lymphoma. Note the scattered vesicles.*

Fig. 13.57 *MRI scan showing progressive multifocal encephalopathy in a patient infected with HIV.*

In HIV-infected patients, as well as in other immunosuppressed patients, such as organ or bone marrow transplant recipients, progressive multifocal leucoencephalopathy (PML or PMLE) may occur in those infected with polyomaviruses. Computed tomography scans of the central nervous system reveal hypodense nonenhancing lesions of white matter (**Fig. 13.57**) whereas MRI scans show signal intensity with T_2-weighted imaging. Progressive dementia frequently occurs in HIV-infected patients. There are currently no proven effective treatment regimens for this infection.

CONCLUSION

Improvements in the management of HIV infection have been dramatic with the advent of more potent antiretroviral drugs, the protease inhibitors. Combination therapy is employed early in the disease to slow the rate of destruction of CD4+ T lymphocytes and to reduce the rate of antiretroviral resistance.

chapter 14

Congenital and Perinatal Infections

INTRODUCTION

The fetus and the neonate behave in many ways as an immunologically impaired host, with increased susceptibility to a variety of viral and bacterial infections, either *in utero* or during the perinatal or neonatal period.

VIRAL INFECTIONS

HERPESVIRUSES

Cytomegalovirus

There are a number of congenitally acquired infections caused by members of the Herpesvirus family. The most common is congenital cytomegalovirus (CMV) infection. Approximately 4000 infants are born in the USA each year with severe congenital CMV syndrome and die in the neonatal period. In its most severe form, the disease is characterized by hepatosplenomegaly, microcephaly, retinitis, intracranial calcifications, petaechiae, thrombocytopenia, direct hyperbilirubinemia and death (**Fig. 14.1**). Plain films of the skull have a characteristic appearance, with periventricular calcifications (**Fig. 14.2**). Another 36,000 congenitally infected infants who survive have complications such as hearing loss, psychomotor delay, retinitis and neurological disease including mental retardation. Primary CMV infection during the first trimester of pregnancy carries the greatest risk of congenital or perinatal disease.

Varicella-zoster virus

Infection in pregnancy with varicella-zoster virus (VZV) can also result in congenital disease. A clinical syndrome of hypoplasia of the extremities, retinitis, cicatricial skin scarring and ocular abnormalities has been described (**Fig. 14.3**). A congenital syndrome may occur in 5% of infants born to mothers who were infected in the first trimester of pregnancy. Neonatal varicella may also occur in infants born to mothers with acute varicella within 4 days of delivery. Administration of varicella-zoster immunoglobulin to neonates exposed to acute infection can prevent this potentially lethal complication.

Herpes simplex virus

Neonatal herpes simplex virus (HSV) infection occurs in 1–2 babies in 5000 deliveries. Typically, presentation occurs between 5 and 17 days after birth. Manifestations vary from disease that is localized to the skin, eyes or mouth to a severe life-threatening encephalitis or involvement of multiple organs. In both disseminated disease and encephalitis, mortality

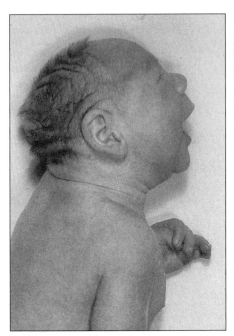

Fig. 14.1 *Child with microcephaly from congenital CMV infection.*

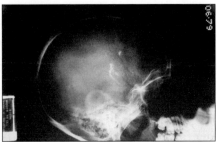

Fig. 14.2 *Plain skull radiograph demonstrating periventricular calcifications typical of congenital CMV infection.*

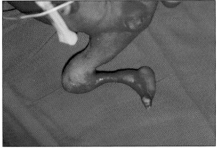

Fig. 14.3 *Hypoplasia of right lower limb in a child with congenital varicella infection.*

can be substantial. Although skin vesicles may be typically present (**Fig. 14.4**), some neonates with disseminated disease do not have any skin lesions. Isolation of HSV from blood, cerebrospinal fluid or skin lesions can serve to make the diagnosis. Direct immunofluorescent staining of skin lesions may also help make a diagnosis. Treatment with intravenous aciclovir reduces the morbidity and mortality.

RUBELLA

Congenital rubella has virtually disappeared owing to adequate levels of childhood immunization. However, fetal disease occurs in about one-half of cases of mothers infected with rubella in the first 2 months of pregnancy. Congenital rubella syndrome is characterized by a variety of ophthalmological manifestations, including cataracts, microphthalmia, glaucoma and retinitis (**Fig. 14.5**). A number of cardiac anomalies, such as patent ductus arteriosus, pulmonary artery stenosis and septal defects, may occur as well. Other central nervous system lesions include sensorineural hearing deficits, microcephaly, meningoencephalitis and mental retardation. Growth retardation, radiolucent bone lesions (**Fig. 14.6**), hepatosplenomegaly, thrombocytopenia, direct hyperbilirubinemia and a purpuric skin rash ('blueberry muffin') caused by extramedullary haematopoiesis may also be noted. Isolation of the virus, the presence of immunoglobulin M antibodies or polymerase chain reaction of the cerebrospinal fluid may enable a diagnosis to be made. Unfortunately there is no effective therapy for congenital rubella infection.

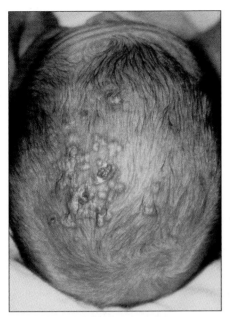

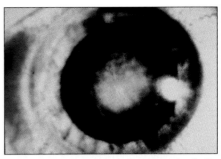

Fig. 14.5 *Cataract from congenital rubella syndrome.*

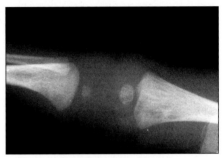

Fig. 14.4 *Vesicles at the site of a scalp electrode in neonatal HSV infection.*

Fig. 14.6 *Radiolucent bone lesions in child with congenital rubella syndrome.*

PARVOVIRUS

Congenital parvovirus infection occurs in approximately 50% of maternal infections. Clinical consequences are largely seen in second trimester infections, when temporary bone marrow aplasia may occur. Fetal anaemia and hydrops fetalis may occur, the most severe outcome being death, although this is rare. Treatment with intrauterine blood transfusions may be necessary. In most cases recovery is complete.

HUMAN IMMUNODEFICIENCY VIRUS

Human immunodeficiency virus (HIV) infection can be transmitted to infants of infected mothers either *in utero*, at the time of delivery or through breast-feeding. The congenital infection is characterized by premature birth or low birth weight. The risk of such vertical transmission can be reduced by antenatal antiretroviral therapy for the mother and treatment of the newborn child in the perinatal period. Increasing evidence suggests that delivery by Caesarian section further reduces the risk, as does avoidance of breast-feeding.

TOXOPLASMOSIS

Toxoplasmosis acquired during pregnancy can lead to development of congenital disease. In contrast to CMV and varicella-zoster infections, transmission is less likely during first trimester; however, if infected, fetal disease is more likely. Congenital toxoplasmosis is

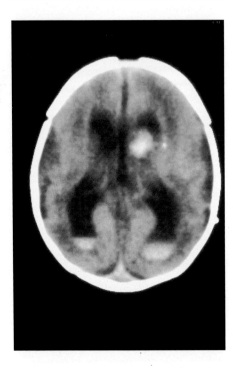

Fig. 14.7 *CT scan demonstrating intracranial calcification in a child with congenital toxoplasmosis.*

manifested by a maculopapular rash, generalized lymphadenopathy, hepatosplenomegaly and thrombocytopenia. Central nervous system involvement can lead to hydrocephaly, microcephaly and retinitis. Intracranial calcification on CT scans also has a characteristic appearance (**Fig. 14.7**). The rate of congenital toxoplasmosis varies throughout the world. Estimates of 1 in 10,000 live births have been made. Diagnosis can be made by polymerase chain reaction or by detection of immunoglobulin M antibodies in the infant. Cerebrospinal fluid characteristically has elevated protein levels and minimal or no cellular reaction.

SYPHILIS

Although congenital syphilis is uncommon, untreated latent maternal disease will result in a congenitally infected infant in 10–20% of cases. Congenital syphilis is generally a multisystem disease. Irregular calcifications of bone, teeth, skin and cartilage may be present. Central nervous system disease, liver failure and pneumonitis may occur. Rapid plasma reagin and specific treponemal antibody absorption studies can be used to screen mothers and monitor infants. Therapy of infected mothers or infants with intravenous penicillin is still the treatment of choice.

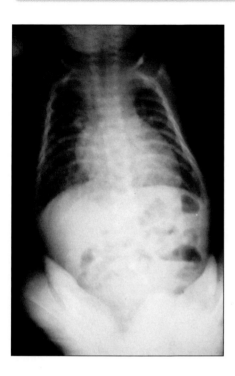

Fig. 14.8 *Chest X-ray of a neonate with* Chlamydia trachomatis *infection.*

OTHER BACTERIA

There are a number of bacterial infections that can complicate pregnancy. *Listeria monocytogenes* can cause both congenital and neonatal syndromes. Infection during early pregnancy may result in fetal death. Other manifestations include bacteraemic multisystem disease with granulomatous infiltration of parenchymal organs. There may be a purplish, nodular rash with hepatosplenomegaly. Neonatal listeriosis occurs after intrapartum exposure and is manifest by bacteraemia and meningitis.

Gonococcal ophthalmia neonatorum may be a complication of birth of an infant to an infected mother. Manifestations include oedema of the eyelids and a purulent exudate associated with swollen conjunctiva. Prophylactic antibiotics administered to the eyes of infants at birth prevents this complication.

Chlamydia trachomatis infection can occur at birth with manifestations of ophthalmia neonatorum. In addition, neonatal pneumonitis may occur at 3–6 weeks of age, causing tachypnoea and repetitive cough. Frank consolidation of lungs on physical examination or chest X-ray (**Fig. 14.8**) may occur. Therapy with erythromycin is curative.

chapter 15

Tropical Infections

INTRODUCTION

Tropical medicine encompasses the management of a wide variety of infectious diseases that are common in tropical climates, some of which, such as tuberculosis and infection with the human immunodeficiency virus (HIV), are also prevalent in temperate countries. However, certain infections are restricted to the tropics, often because of the requirement for certain arthropod vectors like the *Anopheles* mosquito, and are only seen in more temperate regions as imported diseases. This chapter highlights the more important tropical infections and the problems of the returning traveller.

PROTOZOAL INFECTIONS

Protozoan parasites are unicellular organisms many of which have evolved complex life cycles. Unlike helminths, once inside the host protozoa can replicate and multiply rapidly, leading to overwhelming infection. Some of these parasites, such as giardia and amoebae, are usually confined to the gastrointestinal tract but others, such as the causative agents of malaria and leishmaniasis, invade the blood stream, lymphatic vessels or tissues.

MALARIA

Malaria is arguably the world's most important human infection, estimated to cause more than 1 million deaths annually. Four species of *Plasmodium* cause malaria: *Plasmodium falciparum*, *Plasmodium vivax*, *Plasmodium ovale* and *Plasmodium malariae*. Each has its own biological characteristics although the clinical features of malaria can be the same, regardless of which species is involved. *P. falciparum* causes the most severe disease and is responsible for most malaria deaths.

The life cycle of the parasite is shown in **Figure 15.1**. It should be noted that the gametocyte is infective for the mosquito but does not cause symptoms in humans. *P. vivax* and *P. ovale* differ from the other two species in that some of their merozoites may remain dormant in the liver as 'hypnozoites' and may, months or even years later, become activated and reinvade red blood cells to produce clinical relapses.

Malaria is transmitted to humans by the bite of the female *Anopheles* mosquito, which bites at dusk and at night. The disease is widely distributed in the tropics and in the past decade it has spread further as mosquito control has deteriorated (**Fig. 4.8**). The highest rates of malaria transmission occur in coastal western and eastern Africa.

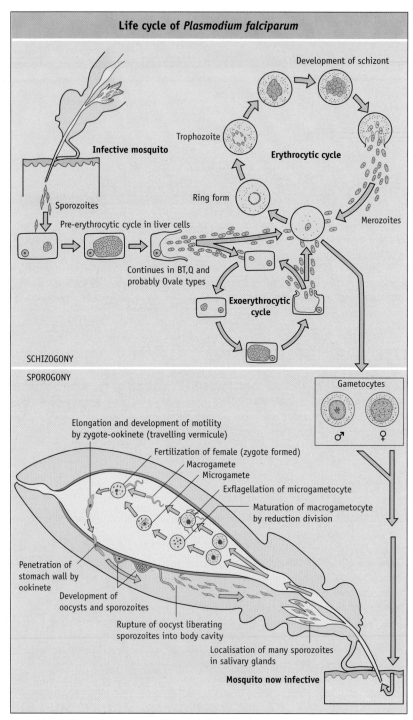

Life cycle of *Plasmodium falciparum*

Development of schizont

Trophozoite

Erythrocytic cycle

Infective mosquito

Ring form

Sporozoites

Merozoites

Pre-erythrocytic cycle in liver cells

Continues in BT,Q and probably Ovale types

Exoerythrocytic cycle

SCHIZOGONY

SPOROGONY

Gametocytes

♂   ♀

Elongation and development of motility by zygote-ookinete (travelling vermicule)

Fertilization of female (zygote formed)

Macrogamete

Microgamete

Exflagellation of microgametocyte

Maturation of macrogametocyte by reduction division

Penetration of stomach wall by ookinete

Development of oocysts and sporozoites

Rupture of oocyst liberating sporozoites into body cavity

Localisation of many sporozoites in salivary glands

Mosquito now infective

Fig. 15.1 *Life cycle of* **Plasmodium falciparum.**

CLINICAL FEATURES

The incubation period from infection to symptoms ranges from 7 days to 18 days but can be as long as 40 days with *P. malariae*. There are no symptoms or signs that are pathognomonic of malaria but a typical attack is characterized by paroxysms of rigors, fevers and sweats, often accompanied by vomiting and sometimes by diarrhoea. These attacks may last up to 12 hours and classically recur every 48 hours in tertian malaria (caused by *P. falciparum*, *P. vivax* and *P. ovale*) and every 72 hours in quartan malaria (caused by *P. malariae*), in synchrony with the release of merozoites from ruptured infected red cells. In practice, such periodicity is not common in falciparum malaria, particularly in nonimmune travellers. Other symptoms include headaches, myalgia and cough. Patients may appear anaemic or jaundiced as a result of haemolysis and they may have splenomegaly.

Falciparum malaria

Malaria due to *P. falciparum* is serious and may be fatal. This parasite can multiply rapidly with the result that a large percentage of the host red cells become parasitized. The clinical features result from a combination of haemolysis, sequestration of parasitized red cells and, probably, cytokine release by the host. In addition to the paroxysms of fever mentioned above, falciparum malaria can cause a variety of complications (**Fig. 15.2**).

The term cerebral malaria refers to unrousable coma secondary to *P. falciparum* when other causes of coma, such as hypoglycaemia, have been excluded (**Fig. 15.3**). Convulsions may occur and there can be prolonged neurological sequelae in survivors, especially children.

Algid malaria is a term used to describe patients with malaria who develop hypotension and shock and become acidotic, often developing acute renal failure.

Blackwater fever is rare and is due to haemoglobinuria and renal failure secondary to brisk haemolysis. The haemolysis occurs after quinine exposure and is immunologically mediated.

Complications of falciparum malaria

Cerebral malaria (unrousable coma)
Severe anaemia
Renal failure
Pulmonary edema
Hypoglycaemia
Cardiovascular collapse, shock ('algid' malaria)
Disseminated intravascular coagulation (DIC)
Repeated generalized seizures
Lactic acidosis
Haemoglobinuria and blackwater fever

Other complications
Impaired consciousness
Prostration; extreme weakness
Hyperparasitaemia
Jaundice
Hyperpyrexia

Fig. 15.2 *Complications of falciparum malaria.*

219

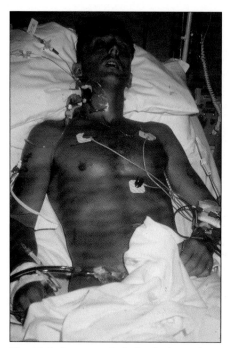

Fig. 15.3 *Severe malaria in the intensive therapy unit.*

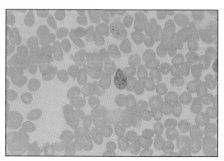

Fig. 15.4 *Thin film of vivax malaria.*

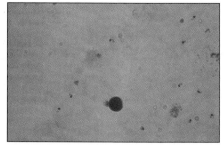

Fig. 15.5 *Thick film showing ring forms of Plasmodium falciparum.*

Vivax malaria

This 'benign tertian malaria' is rarely fatal because the parasitaemia is low grade. The main problems are fever and anaemia. Occasionally, massive splenomegaly occurs and rarely the spleen may rupture spontaneously.

DIAGNOSIS

The differential diagnosis of malaria is wide because the clinical features are nonspecific; the most common misdiagnoses in imported cases are influenza, hepatitis and gastroenteritis. Diagnosis rests on the demonstration of parasites in red blood cells in a blood film (**Fig. 15.4**). Thin films are essential for speciation but thick films are more sensitive for diagnosis (**Fig. 15.5**). It must be emphasized that a single negative film does not exclude the diagnosis of malaria; further films should be made on at least two successive days if the suspicion is strong. Other laboratory findings, such as anaemia, thrombocytopenia and an elevated plasma lactate dehydrogenase are common but nonspecific. Leucocytosis and eosinophilia are not features of malaria.

TREATMENT

Falciparum malaria should be considered a medical emergency and treatment should be instituted as soon as the diagnosis is made. Treatment of malaria caused by the other species is less urgent but still essential. The choice of treatment depends on the species of parasite and the endemic region where the infection was acquired. Chloroquine is still the treatment of choice for vivax, ovale and malariae malaria although some strains of *P. vivax* from the South Pacific are now moderately resistant to chloroquine. Unfortunately, chloroquine resistance in *P. falciparum* is now widespread and resistance to other drugs is increasing, particularly in south-east Asia. Currently, quinine is the 'gold standard' therapy for falciparum malaria. Other drugs that are commonly used are halofantrine, mefloquine and pyrimethamine with sulfadoxine (Fansidar®). The most promising new drug is artemisinine, which is derived from a Chinese herb.

In severe falciparum malaria, supportive treatment is also important to safeguard against hypotension and renal failure, to provide blood products and to prevent hypoglycaemia. Secondary bacterial infections should be sought and treated. The role of exchange transfusion for patients with high-grade parasitaemia is controversial.

Patients who are treated for vivax or ovale malaria should also be given primaquine to eliminate the hepatic 'hypnozoites' and thus prevent relapses. Such patients should have their glucose-6-phosphate dehydrogenase status checked because primaquine can cause haemolysis in those with a deficiency of this enzyme.

CONTROL AND PREVENTION

There is no malarial vaccine although progress in this area looks hopeful. Vector control is essential and the failure to get rid of mosquito breeding sites has led to a resurgence of malaria in many tropical countries. For the individual, trials have shown that the use of pyrmethrin-impregnated mosquito nets provides good protection from malaria. In addition, chemoprophylaxis with drugs such as chloroquine and proguanil (in combination) or with mefloquine can reduce the risk of symptomatic infection in travellers.

TRYPANOSOMIASIS

AFRICAN TRYPANOSOMIASIS

There are two forms of human trypanosomiasis, or sleeping sickness, in Africa caused by subspecies of *Trypanosoma brucei*. An acute form, caused by *T. brucei rhodesiense*, occurs mainly in eastern Africa and is relatively rare. In western Africa, there is a more indolent disease that is caused by *T. brucei gambiense*. Both subspecies of trypanosome are flagellate protozoa that are spread by bite of tsetse flies (*Glossina* spp.), with animal reservoirs of infection that include wild buck and domestic cattle.

The pathogenesis of African trypanosomiasis is poorly understood. There is evidence of lymphocyte activation with high levels of immunoglobulin and circulating immune complexes. The causative organism is capable of rapid antigenic shift by changing its surface proteins, so the host response is evaded.

Clinical features

In both forms of African trypanosomiasis there are usually three stages of infection. Initially after the tsetse bite there is a chancre at the site of inoculation that heals spontaneously within 1 month. Some weeks or months later there is a haemolymphatic stage as the blood stream is invaded; this may manifest as fever, lymphadenopathy or splenomegaly. Enlargement of the posterior cervical lymph nodes (Winterbottom's sign) (**Fig. 15.6**) is common in western African disease. During this second stage, myocarditis and haemolysis may occur. A late, third stage is characterized by a meningoencephalitis with headache and personality changes, later progressing to obvious neurological signs, particularly involving the extrapyramidal system. The disease progresses to coma and death.

Eastern African sleeping sickness is a much more acute and fulminant disease than that seen in the western African form. A fatal meningoencephalitis may develop within a few months of initial infection. In disease due to *T. brucei gambiense* the clinical features may evolve over several years.

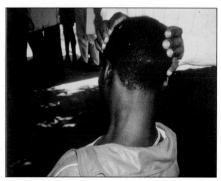

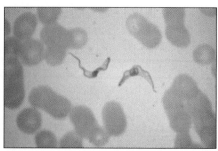

Fig. 15.7 *Blood film showing trypanosome (Trypanosoma brucei rhodesiense).*

Fig. 15.6 *Winterbottom's sign in trypanosomiasis.*

Fig. 15.8 *Morula cell in the cerebrospinal fluid from a patient with sleeping sickness (Trypanosoma brucei gambiense).*

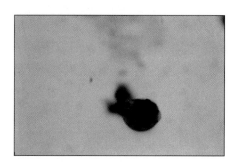

Diagnosis

The diagnosis should be considered in any patient from sub-Saharan Africa with a fever and lymphadenopathy or with unexplained neuropsychological symptoms. Diagnosis rests on the demonstration of the parasite. Thick and thin blood films to find the trypanosomes are particularly useful in eastern African trypanosomiasis (**Fig. 15.7**). The yield can be increased by examining the buffy coat or by sampling bone marrow and lymph node aspirates. Trypanosomes are much more difficult to detect in the western African form of the disease. Indirect evidence of infection includes high serum immunoglobulin levels and the finding of haemolysis. In the meningoencephalitic phase, trypanosomes may be found in the cerebrospinal fluid. There is often a lymphocytosis and raised cerebrospinal fluid protein level. Sometimes morula cells can be found (**Fig. 15.8**).

Treatment

Both forms of disease can be treated with suramin in the first two stages. The drug is given intravenously in weekly doses; however, it has a variety of side effects and is nephrotoxic. Pentamidine is effective against *T. brucei gambiense* but has no activity against the *T. brucei rhodesiense*. Treating the meningoencephalitic stage is difficult. Most experience is with melarsoprol but this drug, too, is toxic. Recently, promising results have been obtained with α-difluoromethylornithine.

Control and prevention

There are no vaccines available but considerable progress has been made in controlling the tsetse fly. Pentamidine has been used as chemoprophylaxis but it is relatively expensive and toxic and may lead to drug-resistant trypanosomes.

SOUTH AMERICAN TRYPANOSOMIASIS

This disease, caused by *Trypanosoma cruzi*, is spread by the triamotid bug. Infective trypomastigotes are shed in the insect faeces and can enter the human host either through damaged skin (e.g. an insect bite) or by contaminating mucous membranes. Infection can also be spread by blood transfusion and, rarely, transplacentally. The disease is confined to the Americas, with most disease in South America, going as far south as the southern parts of Chile and Argentina. There have been occasional case reports from the southern USA.

Clinical features

The parasite is myotropic and most of the serious complications of infection result from muscle damage. As with African trypanosomiasis, the South American disease has three stages. There is an initial lesion at the site of entry of the trypanosome (a chagoma), which is usually near an insect bite or in the mucous membranes. Commonly the mucous membranes of the eye are involved, leading to orbital swelling and a unilateral conjunctivitis (Romaña's sign). After the chagoma, there is an acute phase, which can be mild and go unnoticed. However, fever can occur and is often accompanied by lymphadenopathy, hepatosplenomegaly and a rash. Rarely, in children, an acute myocarditis occurs or there is a potentially fatal meningoencephalitis. The acute phase lasts 1–2 months.

Chronic infection follows and is usually asymptomatic. However, symptomatic disease does occur and usually involves the heart or the gastrointestinal system. Cardiomyopathy with consequent rhythm problems and heart failure may ensue. In the gut there are problems that resemble denervation of the myenteric plexus; mega-oesophagus with dysphagia and malnutrition is more common than megacolon (see **Fig. 9.23**).

Diagnosis

Parasites may be found in blood films or in tissue sections. Serological diagnosis can confirm clinical suspicion in endemic areas. Xenodiagnosis is sometimes used – this involves feeding uninfected triamotid bugs on the patient's blood and then examining the bug's faeces 30–60 days later for evidence of *T. cruzi*.

Treatment

The most promising drugs for treatment are benzonidazole and nifurtimox, which appear to be useful during the acute phase. Chronic disease is managed according to the complications that have occured.

Control and prevention

Control of triamotid bugs, usually through improving housing and house design, is essential in the absence of a vaccine. Screening blood transfusions is also important in endemic areas.

LEISHMANIASIS

Caused by an intracellular protozoan parasite of the genus *Leishmania*, this disease is spread by sandflies. Infected people may develop either cutaneous or visceral disease, although many infections are subclinical. *Leishmania* spp. cannot be distinguished morphologically but can be speciated using molecular methods. They specifically infect cells of the reticuloendothelial system, and the amastigotes may be seen intracellularly with Giemsa staining.

Leishmania species and their distribution

Species	Clinical manifestations	Geographical distribution
Leishmania donovani	Visceral leishmaniasis	Sub-Saharan East Africa, southern Asia, Iran
Leishmania infantum	Visceral leishmaniasis	Mediterranean littoral areas (northern Africa, southern Europe)
Leishmania aethiopica	Cutaneous ulcers, diffuse cutaneous leishmaniasis	Ethiopia and surrounding areas
Leishmania tropica	Cutaneous ulcers, chronic relapsing cutaneous disease	Middle East, southern Asia
Leishmania major	Cutaneous leishmaniasis	Northern Africa, Middle East, southern Asia, central Africa
Leishmania braziliensis complex	Cutaneous leishmaniasis, mucocutaneous disease	Central America to Argentina
Leishmania mexicana complex	Cutaneous leishmaniasis Mucocutaneous disease Diffuse cutaneous disease	Southern USA, Central America, Northern and central South America, Dominican Republic

Fig. 15.9 Leishmania *species and their distribution.*

CUTANEOUS LEISHMANIASIS

This condition is common in the Americas as well as in the Old World and is caused by a variety of species (**Fig. 15.9**). There are animal reservoirs of the parasites, usually rodents and dogs. Transmission can even occur around the Mediterranean littoral.

Clinical features

After an incubation period ranging from 1 week to a few months, a skin lesion appears at the site of the sandfly bite. The initial papule enlarges and ulcerates. The painless ulcer usually has a firm raised edge and a dry crusty centre and there may be smaller satellite lesions nearby (**Fig. 15.10**). Most lesions are self-healing but this may take many months and can leave extensive scars. Certain forms of cutaneous disease do not heal spontaneously:

- diffuse cutaneous leishmaniasis, which is a rare complication of *Leishmania mexicana* and *Leishmania aethiopica* infections and leads to multiple nodules and plaques (without ulceration) that superficially resembles lepromatous leprosy but does not involve nerves;
- leishmaniasis recidivans, which is a rare complication of *Leishmania tropica* that involves new ulcers forming adjacent to almost-healed lesions which, over years, may spread and be locally destructive; and
- American mucocutaneous leishmaniasis (sometimes called espundia), which occurs only with New World species, notably *Leishmania braziliensis*; some time after a skin lesion has healed, a locally destructive mucous membrane lesion arises, usually in the nasopharynx (**Fig. 15.11**).

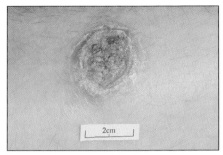

Fig. 15.10 *Typical lesion of cutaneous leishmaniasis.*

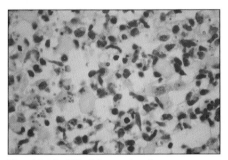

Fig. 15.12 *Skin biopsy showing* Leishmania *amastigotes in macrophages.*

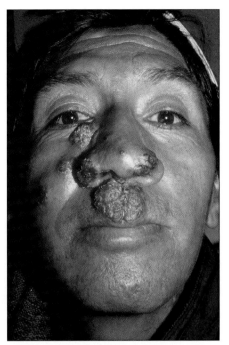

Fig. 15.11 *Mucocutaneous leishmaniasis (espundia) in a man from Ecuador.*

Diagnosis

The diagnosis is suspected with the typical clinical appearances and the appropriate exposure history. The best confirmation is the demonstration of the parasite in the tissues, either by aspiration or biopsy of the ulcer edge (**Fig. 15.12**). Giemsa staining and culture usually yield the diagnosis and speciation can be done using deoxyribonucleic acid probes. In addition there is a delayed hypersensitivity skin test, the leishmanin test, which is often positive in active, ulcerating disease.

Treatment

Because many ulcers are self-healing, the evaluation of treatments can be difficult. Therapy may be local, using heat or cold and single lesions can be curetted or excised. Systemic treatments are used for extensive disease or if *L. braziliensis* is suspected, in order to avoid the development of mucocutaneous disease. The most commonly used systemic treatment is intravenous sodium stibogluconate, given daily for 15–20 days. Other drugs that have been used include pentamidine, amphotericin B, allopurinol and ketoconazole.

VISCERAL LEISHMANIASIS

This condition is widespread but is most commonly seen in the Indian subcontinent and in Africa. Although sandflies are the principal vectors, the infection can be transmitted via blood transfusions. The parasite spreads throughout the body following inoculation without the formation of a skin lesion in most cases. After an incubation period of a few months, the disease begins insidiously with fever, weight loss and weakness. Typical signs include lymphadenopathy and hepatosplenomegaly with fever (**Fig. 15.13**). Without treatment most cases progress inexorably to cachexia and death, often from secondary infections.

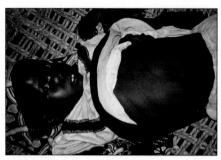

Fig. 15.13 *Hepatosplenomegaly in visceral leishmaniasis.*

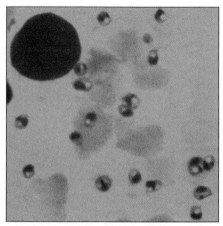

Fig. 15.14 *Bone marrow showing* Leishmania *in visceral leishmaniasis.*

Diagnosis may be suspected with the above clinical features but should be confirmed by finding the parasite. The tissues with the best yield are the buffy coat, bone marrow (**Fig. 15.14**), lymph nodes and spleen. Splenic aspirates are safe and reliable in experienced hands. Serological tests have good sensitivity and specificity. However, the leishmanin skin test is negative and there is general anergy to other skin tests. In addition, there is often a mild pancytopenia and marked hypergammaglobulinaemia.

It should be noted that visceral leishmaniasis may occur in patients with HIV infection who have visited endemic areas. Because of poor cell-mediated immunity, disseminated disease may occur in these patients even when infected with species that normally cause only cutaneous leishmaniasis.

Treatment is with sodium stibogluconate but resistance may occur. Newer approaches include the use of liposomal amphotericin B.

CONTROL AND PREVENTION

There are no vaccines against leishmaniasis so vector control is important as is the removal of animal reservoirs such as rodents.

HELMINTH INFECTIONS

Worms are grouped into three main phyla;
- annelids;
- platyhelminths.
- nematodes

The only annelids of medical interest are leeches, which have a long history of use by doctors and are currently used to reduce wound haematomas after plastic surgery. Occasionally, this practice may lead to wound infections as some leeches carry bacteria such as *Aeromonas* spp. Nematodes, or roundworms, that affect humans live either in the gastrointestinal tract or in the blood or lymphatic vessels. The platyhelminths, or flatworms, are subdivided into two classes:
- trematodes, or flukes, such as *Schistosoma mansoni*, always have a mollusc as their first intermediate host;

- cestodes, or tapeworms, have a head (scolex) and segmented body and live in the gut of the infected host.

Worms are metazoans and are more complex organisms than protozoan parasites, eliciting more of a host response. As the worms migrate through tissues, part of the host response is an eosinophilia, a feature not seen in protozoan infections. Also, unlike the protozoa, worms do not multiply within the human host and must leave the host to reproduce. Therefore, heavy worm infections can only result from recurrent exposure whereas overwhelming protozoan infections can arise from rapid multiplication of a single infecting organism.

NEMATODES

FILARIAL INFECTIONS

There are four important filarial infections that affect humans in the tropics. Two (*Wuchereria bancrofti* and *Brugia malayi*) are lymphatic filaria and the others (*Onchocerci volvulus* and *Loa loa*) are nonlymphatic.

Although each is different, they share certain features, particularly in terms of life cycles. All are transmitted by arthropod vectors (**Fig. 15.15**). The bite of the arthropod transmits an infective larva that slowly matures over some months into a mature adult worm that inhabits the lymphatics or subcutaneous tissues. The adults may live for several years and produce microfilariae, which may survive in the host for up to 2 years. The microfilariae cannot develop further in humans but may be taken up by the appropriate vector when it next bites. In endemic areas, infected people often have no evidence of clinical disease. The development of symptoms depends on the intensity of infection, or the number of adult worms and microfilariae that accumulate in the host.

Lymphatic filariasis

Bancroftian filariasis is the most widespread human filarial infection and is found throughout the tropics, while brugian filariasis is restricted to Asia. In both cases, transmission is by night-biting mosquitos, so the parasites have a nocturnal periodicity.

Clinical features

These infections may present acutely with fever and enlarged regional lymph glands or there may be chronic presentation with lymphatic obstruction and oedema (**Fig. 15.16**). Rarely, in severe cases, elephantiasis results. Bancroftian infections involve the lymphatics of the genitalia so men may present acutely with epididymo-orchitis or chronically with varicocoeles. Neither of these features occur in brugian disease. Lymphoedema of the limbs is limited to either below the knee or below the elbow.

Filaria and their arthropod vectors

Species	Vector	Periodicity
Wucheria bancrofti	Mosquito	Nocturnal
Brugia malayi	Mosquito	Nocturnal
Onchocerca volvulus	Blackfly	None
Loa loa	Horsefly	Diurnal
Mansonella spp.	Midges	None

Fig. 15.15 *Filaria and their arthropod vectors.*

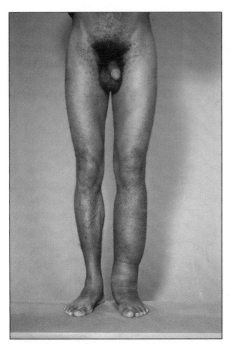

Fig. 15.16 *Oedema and lymph nodes in filariasis.*

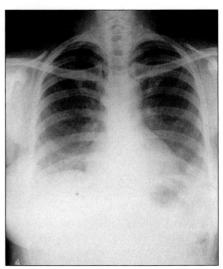

Fig. 15.17 *Chest X-ray showing pulmonary infiltrates in tropical eosinophilia.*

Fig. 15.18 *Microfilaria in blood film.*

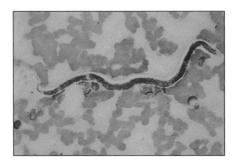

Both species may lead to tropical pulmonary eosinophilia as parasites migrate through the lungs. This is characterised by cough, fever, shortness of breath and patchy infiltrates on the chest X-ray (**Fig. 15.17**). There is an accompanying peripheral blood eosinophilia. This syndrome is usually only seen in India and south-east Asia.

Diagnosis
Although it can be suspected clinically, the diagnosis should be confirmed by demonstrating microfilaria in blood films. Blood is best obtained at night, near midnight, because of the parasite periodicity. Thick and thin films should be examined (**Fig. 15.18**). Microfilariae may also be seen in lymph node aspirates.

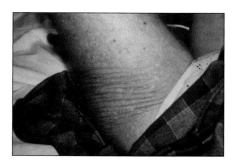

Fig. 15.19 *Skin appearance in chronic onchocerciasis.*

Treatment

The standard treatment has been diethylcarbamazine, which kills microfilariae and will kill most adult worms. More than one course may be required and some patients have reactions a few hours after treatment owing to the death of microfilariae. There is often headache, fever and myalgia. More recently, a newer drug, ivermectin, has been shown to be effective. However, for chronic disease, drugs are of limited benefit and pressure bandages or surgery may be required for symptoms.

Control and prevention

Chemoprophylaxis and vaccines are not available, so control rests with vector control and limiting exposure.

ONCHOCERCIASIS

Transmitted by black flies that inhabit forests near fast-flowing streams, onchocerciasis is particularly common in western Africa but it also occurs in Latin America and even in the Yemen. The adult worms may reach 50cm in length and live in nodules in subcutaneous tissue. However, most of the clinical problems are caused by microfilariae.

Clinical features

Nodules, skin lesions and eye lesions are the common manifestations of onchocerciasis. The nodules are caused by adult worms and are often palpable even though they are deep in the tissues. Nodules on the head are more commonly associated with eye problems. Skin lesions usually overly nodules and are caused by microfilariae. There is usually an intense itch, and scratching leads to excoriation and secondary infection. Chronic disease leads to lichenification and hypopigmentation (**Fig. 15.19**). Eye disease ('river blindness') is a particular feature of disease in western Africa and is rare elsewhere. Microfilariae invade the eye and can affect any structure other than the lens, causing anything from a mild keratitis to a severe choroidoretinitis.

Diagnosis

Diagnosis rests on demonstrating microfilariae in the skin or eye. Skin snips are obtained from involved skin and examined in saline under the dissecting microscope for motile microfilariae. Slit lamp examination may reveal intraocular microfilariae. Nodules may be able to be excised to reveal the adult worm. Sometimes, a provocative test (the Mazotti test) is used: diethylcarbamazine is given in a small dose (50mg) and in a positive test, intense itching and an exacerbation of the rash occur within 24 hours.

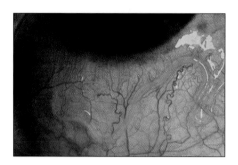

Fig. 15.20 Loa loa *filaria migrating across the conjunctiva.*

Treatment

Diethylcarbamazine is effective against microfilariae but it does not kill the adult worms. Suramin kills the adults but is quite toxic. Over the past decade, ivermectin has become the treatment of choice for onchocerciasis and is now used in mass treatment programs. Sometimes, excision of nodules on the head is advised to reduce the risk of eye disease.

Control and prevention

Vector control is important but recently periodic mass treatment of villages in endemic areas has led to a reduction in infections and in eye disease.

LOA LOA

Loa loa is found only in the forests of western and central Africa and is transmitted by *Chrysops* flies. The adult worms are long-lived and, unlike the adults of onchocerciasis, they are freely mobile in subcutaneous tissues. The microfilariae live up to 1 year but cause little host damage. They have a diurnal periodicity in keeping with the daytime biting habits of *Chrysops* flies.

Clinical features

The adult takes about 5 months to develop after an infecting bite. Migration of the adult causes itching and myalgia and is associated with transient oedematous subcutaneous lumps, called Calabar swellings. Rarely, the patient may notice a worm migrating through the tissues or even across the conjunctivae (**Fig. 15.20**).

Diagnosis

The clinical features are characteristic with the correct geographical exposure history. Microfilariae may be demonstrated in daytime blood films.

Treatment

Diethylcarbamazine is effective against adults and microfilariae although reactions may be seen in heavy infections. Ivermectin is also effective.

Control and prevention

Fly control and appropriate clothing reduce the risk of bites. There is some evidence that monthly chemoprophylaxis with diethylcarbamazine is effective.

OTHER TISSUE NEMATODES

Other tissue nematodes are listed in **Figure 15.21**

Tissue nematodes			
Species	**How contracted**	**Tissue involved**	**Geographical distribution**
Dracunculus medinensis (guineaworm)	By drinking water that contains small crustacea (*Cyclops*)	Subcutaneous tissue	Africa/South Asia
Trichinella spiralis	By eating meat of carnivorous animals	Striated muscle	Widespread
Toxocara canis	By ingesting contaminated soil	Eye, many other tissues	Widespread

Fig. 15.21 *Tissue nematodes.*

INTESTINAL NEMATODES

Intestinal nematodes do not have an intermediate vector but are passed from human to human via faecally excreted eggs or larvae that develop in soil under certain conditions and then become infectious.

ASCARIS LUMBRICOIDES

This large roundworm is the most prevalent roundworm in the tropics, largely because the female produces huge numbers of eggs and the eggs are resistant to environmental factors. Most infections occur in Asia and predominantly affect children. The worm lives in the small intestine, with numerous eggs being shed in the faeces. Ingested eggs in contaminated food (or from dirty hands) hatch in the jejunum into larvae, which penetrate the bowel wall and migrate to the liver. Developing larvae travel to the lungs, then to the trachea and eventually reach the small bowel by tracking into the pharynx and down the oesophagus.

Clinical features

Most infections are asymptomatic but when symptoms occur, they relate either to the passage of larvae through the lungs or to worms in the intestine. The pulmonary symptoms of shortness of breath, cough and wheeze in association with an eosinophilia and chest X-ray infiltrates is known as Loeffler's syndrome. In the abdomen, there may be pain or diarrhoea and, sometimes, a worm may be vomited. Rarely, very heavy worm infections may lead to bowel obstruction.

Diagnosis

This is usually made by finding eggs in the stool or by identifying a worm that has been expelled (see **Figs 15.22** and **9.21**).

Treatment

A variety of broad-spectrum antihelminthic drugs are effective, including piperazine, pyrantel palmoate and mebendazole.

HOOKWORM

There are two main species of hookworm that affect humans: *Ancylostoma duodenale* and *Necator americanus*. The adult worms inhabit the small intestine, shedding numerous eggs

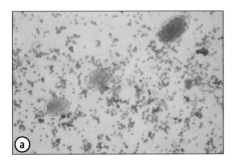

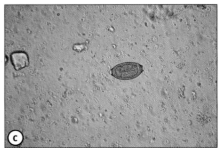

Fig. 15.22 *Helminth ova (a)* Ascaris lumbricoides *(b)* Enterobias *(c)* Trichuris.

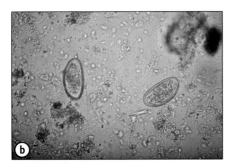

Fig. 15.23 *Hookworm in the gut.*

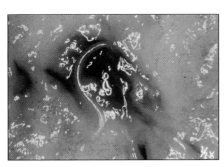

into the faeces. The eggs hatch within 24 hours of excretion into larvae, which gradually change into infective forms that penetrate the skin (usually of the foot). The larvae then enter the circulation and migrate via the lungs, trachea and oesophagus to reach the small intestine where they mature into adult worms (**Fig. 15.23**). *N. americanus* can live up to 5 years whereas *A. duodenale* survives in the host for only 1 year.

Clinical features

The presence of symptoms reflects the worm burden of the individual. As the worms 'grip' the intestinal mucosa they cause slight bleeding, so the most common problem is an iron deficiency anaemia, which may become pronounced during pregnancy. Very occasionally, the passage of larvae through the tissues may cause a hypersensitivity reaction, visceral larva migrans, that resembles Loeffler's syndrome.

Diagnosis

This usually depends on finding the characteristic eggs in the stool. Rarely, worms may be seen on endoscopy or at surgery.

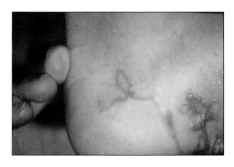

Fig. 15.24 *Foot showing a cutaneous larva migrans rash.*

Treatment

Mebendazole or pyrantel palmoate are effective and are best given as two courses separated by 2 weeks. In addition, anaemia should be corrected with iron therapy.

CUTANEOUS LARVA MIGRANS

Humans may be infected by nonhuman hookworms, such as *Ancylostoma braziliense*. In these cases, the larvae penetrate the skin but cannot reach the circulation. Instead, they migrate through the dermis and travel around deeper tissues, exciting a tissue reaction and causing a serpiginous, erythematous rash (**Fig. 15.24**). This 'creeping eruption' can be intensely itchy. It will resolve over a period of weeks or months as the larvae eventually die. Thiabendazole or albendazole lead to rapid resolution of symptoms.

STRONGYLOIDIASIS

Strongyloides stercoralis, or threadworm, is potentially the most serious nematode infection. This is because autoinfection can occur (unlike the situation in other worm infections), leading to long-lasting infection. The worm life cycle is extremely complex (**Fig. 15.25**), but essentially the larvae can be free-living in the soil and infect by skin penetration or, in certain conditions, infective filariform larvae can develop in the host's perianal region. In this latter case, the larvae can re-enter the circulation and sustain infection. Humans are the main reservoir of *S. stercoralis* but dogs and cats can sometimes harbour this worm.

Clinical features

Infection can be acute, chronic or can lead to hyperinfection.

Acute infection

After skin penetration there may follow a rapidly moving urticarial rash (larva currens), which is most commonly found on the thighs and buttocks in cases of autoinfection (**Fig. 15.26**). Loeffler's syndrome may also occur during larval migration. Afterwards, gastrointestinal symptoms such as pain, nausea or diarrhoea may feature.

Chronic infection

Persisting infections characterized by intermittent cutaneous or gastrointestinal symptoms can occur. These have been best described in Second World War prisoners of war in the Far East.

Hyperinfection

This is a serious complication in those with chronic infection who become immunosuppressed by corticosteroids, cancer or malnutrition. It also occurs in human

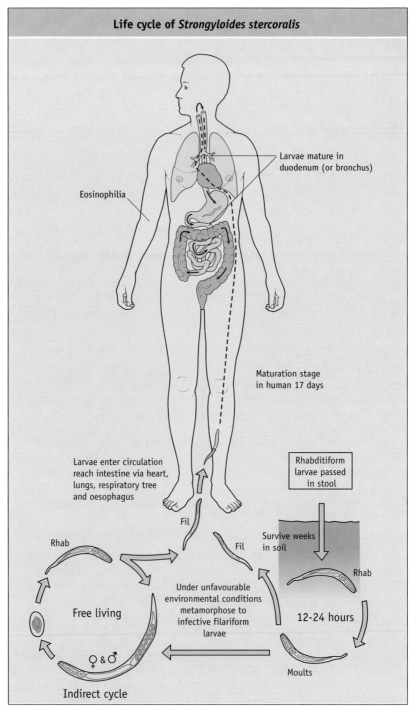

Fig. 15.25 *Life cycle of* Strongyloides stercoralis. *Rhab = rhabditiform larvae; Fil = filariform larvae.*

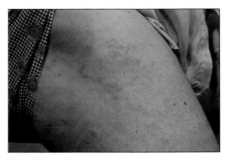

Fig. 15.26 *Rash of larva currens on the thigh in strongyloidiasis.*

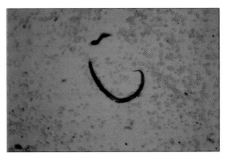

Fig. 15.27 *Strongyloides larva in sputum in hyperinfection case.*

immunodeficiency virus (HIV) infection, but this is remarkably rare. With loss of cell-mediated immunity, larvae rapidly disseminate to many organs, including the central nervous system. Extensive bowel perforation by the migrating larvae frequently leads to Gram-negative bacterial sepsis. Larvae that enter the central nervous system may take bacteria with them, causing Gram-negative bacterial meningitis. Eosinophilia is rare in cases of hyperinfection. Mortality approaches 90%.

Diagnosis
Clinical suspicion is required, especially in cases of hyperinfection. Larvae should be sought in the stool or by duodenal biopsy or aspirate. In hyperinfection, larvae may be found elsewhere, such as in the sputum (**Fig. 15.27**).

Treatment
Thiabendazole is the treatment of choice. It is usually given for 3 days and repeated a week later. Albendazole may also be effective.

WHIPWORM AND PINWORM
Trichuris trichuria (whipworm) and *Enterobius vermicularis* (pinworm) are widely distributed, confined to humans and, unlike the other intestinal nematodes described above, do not migrate through the tissues. The adult worms of both species live in the caecum and ascending colon. Ingested eggs hatch into larvae in the small bowel and mature over a few months, settling in the caecum. Female whipworms shed eggs into the faeces but the female pinworm migrates to the anus, where she deposits eggs.

Clinical features
Most infections are asymptomatic but occasionally abdominal pain or diarrhoea occur. The most common symptom in pinworm infection is perianal pruritis following egg deposition, and secondary bacterial infection may arise in excoriated perineal skin.

Diagnosis
Whipworm can be diagnosed by finding the characeristic 'tea-tray' eggs in the stool (see **Fig. 15.22c**). Pinworm eggs are easily detected by means of the 'cellotape test.' Sellotape is stuck around the anus in the morning before defecating or bathing. Deposited eggs will stick to the tape and can be transferred on the tape to a microscope slide for identification (**Fig. 15.28**). Eggs may be found in the stool and sometimes worms may be seen on colonoscopy.

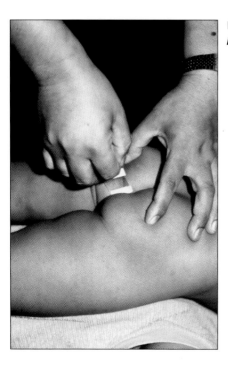

Fig. 15.28 *Positive sellotape test for pinworm eggs.*

Intestinal nematodes
Ascaris lumbricoides *Ancylostoma duodenales* (hookworm) *Necator americanus* (hookworm) *Strongyloides stercoralis* *Trichuris trichuria* (whipworm) *Enterobius vermicularis* (pinworm)

Fig. 15.29 *Intestinal nematodes.*

Treatment
Mebendazole or albendazole are effective against whipworm. Pinworm can be treated with mebendazole, piperazine or pyrantel palmoate.

OTHER INTESTINAL NEMATODES
These are listed in **Figure 15.29**.

CESTODES

TAENIA SAGINATA AND *TAENIA SOLIUM*
Taenia saginata (beef tapeworm) and *Taenia solium* (pork tapeworm) are acquired by eating undercooked, infested meat, although infection can also occur from ingestion of food contaminated with larvae. The adult worm can reach up to 10m in length (in the case of *T. saginata*) and 8m (in the case of *T. solium*). *T. saginata*, has humans as its only definitive host but *T. solium* can develop in a variety of species.

Clinical features
Most patients are unaware of being infected though some may have vague abdominal discomfort. Infection comes to light when the person passes tapeworm segments (proglottids) and sees them in the stool. There may be perianal discomfort when proglottids are passed.

Diagnosis
Infections may be accompanied by a mild eosinophilia and raised serum immunoglobulin E. There are no useful serological tests. Examination of stool specimens for proglottids or eggs is essential. The proglottids of these two species can be distinguished morphologically whereas the eggs cannot (**Fig. 15.30**).

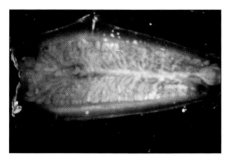

Fig. 15.30 *Proglottid of* Taenia saginata.

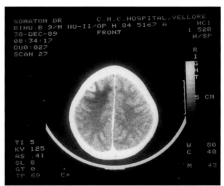

Fig. 15.31 *MRI scan of cerebral cysticercosis.*

Treatment

The treatment of choice is praziquantel as a single dose. Niclosamide is also effective.

Prevention

These infections can be avoided by the proper inspection and cooking of meat.

CYSTICERCOSIS

This condition results from the human ingestion of the larval stages of *T. solium*. It usually follows the consumption of undercooked pork but it may result from autoinfection with eggs from the tapeworm or from hatched eggs contaminating food. Cysticercosis is particularly common in Latin America. Hatched eggs penetrate the small bowel and are disseminated by the bloodstream to various organs where they grow into small, fluid-filled cysticerci. Clinical features result from the presence of these cysticerci.

Clinical features

It usually takes several years for the disseminating cysticerci to produce symptoms. The most common site of these lesions is the brain and, thus, seizures are the most common clinical manifestation. Patients may also present with raised intracranial pressure or with psychiatric illness. Cysticerci may lead to pressure symptoms in the spinal cord as well. Ocular cysticercosis is relatively common and may cause anything from iritis to retinal detachment. Elsewhere in the body, lesions are rarely symptomatic but may be incidental findings.

Diagnosis

Definitive diagnosis is made by demonstrating the parasite in histological sections of affected tissue. However, the constellation of symptoms, findings on CT scans or MRI scans (Fig. 15.31), serology and an eosinophilia should make the diagnosis of neurocysticercosis certain, particularly if there is a good exposure history.

Treatment

The parasite is susceptible to praziquantel and to albendazole; the combination of these drugs is favoured by some experts. In acute infections, killing of the parasite may lead to severe inflammatory reactions. Thus chemotherapy is contraindicated for ocular disease and may need to be covered by dexamethasone in the case of neurocysticercosis. Surgery may be required for some cases.

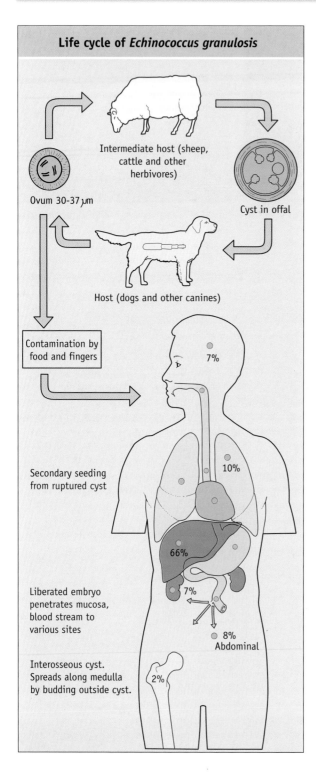

Fig. 15.32 *Life cycle of Echinococcus granulosis.*

Life cycle of *Echinococcus granulosis*

Intermediate host (sheep, cattle and other herbivores)

Ovum 30-37 μm

Cyst in offal

Host (dogs and other canines)

Contamination by food and fingers

7%

Secondary seeding from ruptured cyst

10%

66%

Liberated embryo penetrates mucosa, blood stream to various sites

7%

8% Abdominal

Interosseous cyst. Spreads along medulla by budding outside cyst.

2%

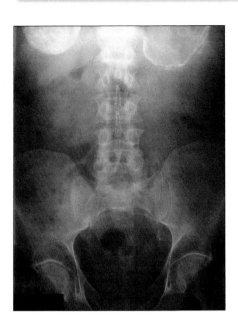

Fig. 15.33 *Plain abdominal X-ray showing calcified hydatid cysts in the spleen and liver.*

ECHINOCOCCOSIS

Echinococcosis (hydatid disease) is a zoonosis that affects humans when they are infected with the larval stage of the dog tapeworm, *Echinococcus granulosus*. This worm requires two hosts (**Fig. 15.32**). It lives in the dog intestine and its eggs are excreted, often in large numbers, in the dog's faeces. Animals, particularly sheep, that graze on contaminated pasture, develop larval cysts in their livers and lungs. Dogs are reinfected by eating infected offal but humans can be incidentally infected by contamination of food or hands with dog faeces. The human then develops cysts in the liver and lungs (and sometimes in other organs) when the eggs hatch and larvae migrate through the intestine into lymphatic vessels and the portal tract.

Clinical features

Most human infections are asymptomatic and cysts are discovered incidentally. The majority of cysts are in the liver and symptoms arise as a result of pressure effects; the cysts sometimes cause pain and occasionally lead to obstructive jaundice. Lung cysts may cause cough or haemoptysis. If cysts are ruptured accidentally, spillage of the contents may lead to peritonitis or pleurisy and, occasionally, to allergic reactions including anaphylaxis.

Diagnosis

Cysts may be identified by a variety of radiological techniques and characteristically contain 'daughter cysts' and hydatic sand (**Fig. 15.33**). Serological tests are about 90% sensitive but the Casoni skin test is no longer used. Cysts may be confirmed histologically in surgical specimens.

Treatment

Until relatively recently, surgery was the only way of removing hydatid cysts. More recently, chemotherapy with a combination of albendazole and praziquantel has yielded good results, sometimes as an adjunct to surgery. The majority of cysts require no treatment as there are no symptoms.

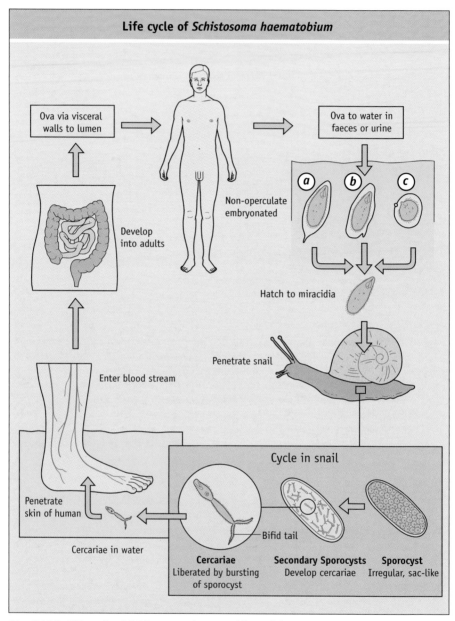

Life cycle of *Schistosoma haematobium*

Ova via visceral
walls to lumen

Ova to water in
faeces or urine

Non-operculate
embryonated

(a)   (b)   (c)

Develop
into adults

Hatch to miracidia

Penetrate snail

Enter blood stream

Cycle in snail

Penetrate
skin of human

Bifid tail

Cercariae in water

Cercariae
Liberated by bursting
of sporocyst

Secondary Sporocysts
Develop cercariae

Sporocyst
Irregular, sac-like

Fig. 15.34 *Life cycle of* Schistosoma haematobium. *(a)* S. haematobium;
(b) S. mansoni; *(c)* S. japonicum.

Prevention

Education programmes promoting good hygiene for dog owners and mass treatment of
infected dogs have led to a decline in hydatid disease in some areas, such as Australia.

TREMATODES OR FLUKES

SCHISTOSOMIASIS

Schistosomiasis, or bilharzia, is the most common human fluke infection and is caused by three main species: *Schistosoma haematobium*, *Schistosoma mansoni* and *Schistosoma japonicum*. The first two are widely distributed in the tropics in Africa, Asia and the Middle East whereas *S. japonicum* is found in the Far East. There is a complex life cycle involving snails, fresh water and humans (**Fig. 15.34**). Infective cercariae penetrate intact human skin, larvae migrate through the lungs and eventually adult worms settle, usually in the mesenteric venous plexus, mate and produce millions of eggs. The eggs are distributed by the venous system, usually to the liver (in the case of *S. mansoni*) or the bladder (in the case of *S. haematobium*). Host reaction to the eggs leads to pathological and clinical sequelae.

Clinical features

The consequences of infection with schistosomes can be divided into acute, allergic and chronic diseases. After contact with fresh water, some patients get a dermatitis ('swimmer's itch') as the infective cercariae penetrate the skin. Some weeks later, some people have an acute, allergic reaction to the parasite that presents with fever, rigors and a marked eosinophilia. This reaction is called Katayama fever and is most common in infections with *S. japonicum*.

Chronic problems are more common and result from the granulomatous reaction to deposited eggs. The liver and the intestinal tract are primarily affected with *S. mansoni* and *S. japonicum* whereas *S. haematobium* affects the genitourinary system. Granuloma formation in the liver may lead to hepatic fibrosis and subsequent portal hypertension with its myriad consequences. In the gut, diarrhoea may result and polyps may form secondary to the granulomata and may mimic carcinoma or Crohn's disease. Bladder involvement may cause urinary frequency or haematuria. Over time, secondary bacterial infections may be a problem as the bladder mucosa becomes more abnormal and, in some endemic areas, squamous cell carcinoma of the bladder results from chronic inflammation. Rarely, other tissues, such as the brain, spinal cord and lungs may be the sites of egg deposition.

Diagnosis

Schistosomiasis may be suspected epidemiologically from a travel history and symptoms. Eggs can often be demonstrated in the urine or stools or from bladder biopsies and rectal snips (**Fig. 15.35**). Serology using an enzyme-linked immunosorbent assay based on egg antigens can be useful in areas where the disease is not endemic. Eosinophilia is a common but nonspecific finding.

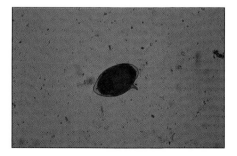

Fig. 15.35 **Schistosoma mansoni** *ova in stool.*

Flukes that affect humans

Species	Site of infection	Vehicle	Geographical distribution
Liver flukes			
Opisthorchis viverrini	Bile ducts	Raw fish	South-East Asia
Clonorchis sinensis	Bile ducts	Raw fish	Far East
Fasciola hepatica	Bile ducts	Watercress	Widespread
Lung flukes			
Paragonimus westermani	Lung	Freshwater crab	Far East, West Africa, South America
Intestinal flukes			
Fasciola buski	Jejunum	Aquatic plants	Far East
Echinostoma spp.	Small bowel	Fish	Far East
Gastroduodenalis hominis	Caecum	Plants	Southern Asia

Fig. 15.36 *Flukes that affect humans.*

Treatment

All *Schistosoma* spp. respond to praziquantel, which is now the treatment of choice. Other drugs include oxamniquine for *S. mansoni* infection and metrifonate for *S. haematobium* infection.

Prevention

There are, as yet, no vaccines, so disease control rests on mass treatment programmes of infected individuals along with snail control and improvements in hygiene and water safety.

OTHER FLUKES

A variety of other flukes affect humans in a variety of settings (**Fig. 15.36**). The common features are that the life cycles of these parasites involve fresh water and some sort of mollusc as an intermediate host. The flukes may lodge in the intestine, the liver or the lungs and the clinical problems they cause relate to the organ sytem they inhabit.

BACTERIAL INFECTIONS IN THE TROPICS

Although bacterial pneumonia, meningitis and sepsis are all common causes of morbidity and mortality in the tropics, other conditions are acquired only in the tropics and subtropics but may be imported to temperate regions.

TYPHOID

Enteric fever due to *Salmonella typhi* and to *Salmonella paratyphi* A and B is common in the tropics. These bacteria are spread by the faecal–oral route and lead to systemic disease, often with early gastrointestinal symptoms. Further details may be found in Chapter 9.

RELAPSING FEVER

Relapsing fever is caused by a spirochaete of the *Borrelia* genus. This condition is found throughout the tropics but it may also occur in temperate regions. In louse-borne relapsing fever, humans act as the reservoir whereas in tick-borne disease, rodents form the main

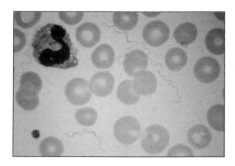

Fig. 15.37 *Blood film showing* **Borrelia** *spirochaetes.*

reservoir of infection. The louse-borne disease is particularly common in northern Africa and Ethiopia and Sudan and may occur in epidemics when conditions favour infestations of body lice. Tick-borne relapsing fever is usually sporadic and more widely spread globally. In either case, an infected arthropod bites the human and inoculates the *Borrelia* spirochaete into the lymphatics or blood stream.

Clinical features

Borrelia spp. do not secrete any toxins and most features of the disease are secondary to cytokine release as part of the host defences. Symptoms resemble severe influenza with myalgia, headache, fever and a dry cough. There may be a petaechial skin rash and hepatosplenomegaly. In severe cases, disseminated intravascular coagulation may be seen.

Diagnosis

Diagnosis may be entirely based on clinical findings during outbreaks, but definite diagnosis relies on the finding of spirochaetes in blood smears (**Fig. 15.37**).

Treatment

Most cases resolve without specific treatment but tetracyclines or macrolides are the treatments of choice. In louse-borne relapsing fever particularly, treatment may result in a Jarisch–Herxheimer reaction. This may be prevented by adequate hydration and pretreatment with a nonsteroidal anti-inflammatry drug such as ibuprofen.

RICKETTSIAL INFECTIONS

Rickettsia are small, intracellular bacteria that are transmitted to humans by the bites of various arthropod vectors. Various species occur throughout the world and infections either lead to a 'spotted fever' or to typhus. Q fever is a particular zoonotic infection due to *Coxiella burnetii* and is biologically distinct from the other rickettsial infections. Rickettsial infections vary in severity but most are acute, self-limiting febrile illnesses.

Rocky Mountain spotted fever is the most severe rickettsial infection. It produces a severe vasculitis that may lead to disseminated intravascular coagulation, shock and death. Scrub typhus, which is limited to the Far East, may also be severe. However, most imported disease in the West is due to African tick typhus (fièvre boutonneuse), which is caused by *Rickettsia conorii*. This is usually a mild flu-like illness, although the myalgia may be quite severe. There is often a mild, macular rash (**Fig. 15.38**) and careful examination usually reveals the eschar, the site of the inoculating tick bite (**Fig. 15.39**).

Diagnosis

The diagnosis is often clinical but it can often be confirmed with specific rickettsial serology. Rarely, organisms may be isolated from blood in the first week of illness.

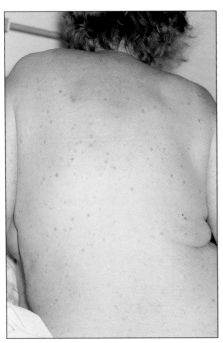

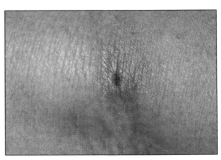

Fig. 15.39 *Eschar at site of tick bite.*

Fig. 15.38 *Skin rash in African tick typhus.*

Treatment

Many cases are self-limiting but supportive therapy is required for severe cases. Tetracyclines or chloramphenicol are active against rickettsiae and the use of either will lead to an earlier resolution of symptoms.

LEPROSY

Leprosy (Hansen's disease) results from infection with *Mycobacterium leprae*, an organism that is extremely slow growing and cannot be cultured *in vitro*. Instead, cultures are made in mouse foot pads and in the tail of the nine-banded armadillo. *M. leprae* is probably spread from human to human via respiratory droplets; infectious people have numerous bacilli in the nasal mucosa. Infectivity is low and it may take many years for symptoms to develop. Most of the clinical features of leprosy result from damage to skin, the eyes and peripheral nerves. Leprosy bacilli grow best at temperatures somewhat below body temperature, and hence peripheral nerves and exposed skin are the sites of predeliction.

CLINICAL FEATURES

The clinical problems associated with leprosy depend critically on the host immune response to the infecting bacilli.

Tuberculoid disease

When cell-mediated immunity is good, paucibacillary or tuberculoid leprosy results. In patients with tuberculoid disease, presentation is frequently due to peripheral nerve lesions, such as ulnar palsy, resulting from granuloma formation around the nerve. Skin lesions, if present, are usually solitary although occasionally two or three plaques may be present. These

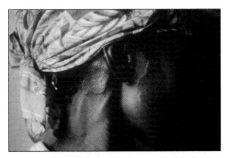

Fig. 15.40 *Thickened nerve and skin lesion in tuberculoid leprosy.*

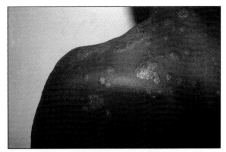

Fig. 15.41 *Numerous skin lesions in lepromatous leprosy.*

skin lesions are often scaly, have no hair growth and diminished sweating and are usually partially anaesthetic. There may be thickened nerves in the area of the plaque (**Fig. 15.40**).

Lepromatous leprosy

When cell-mediated immunity is poor or absent, bacilli multiply easily. In multibacillary, or lepromatous, disease, nasal stuffiness may be an early symptom. Skin lesions are frequent and numerous; they may be macules, papules or nodules. Macules tend to appear first. Nerve involvement is a late feature and therefore patients with multibacillary disease, who are the most infectious, unfortunately often present late. Lesions may be copper-coloured on dark skin (**Fig. 15.41**). As the disease progresses, affected skin becomes indurated; on the face this gives rise to the 'leonine' appearance. Nerve thickening also occurs late, as does a symmetrical glove and stocking sensory neuropathy. This neuropathy in turn leads to tissue damage in anaesthetic limbs. Nasal damage from bacillary growth may cause collapse of the nasal bridge. An iritis may also occur.

Borderline leprosy

The most common type of leprosy occurs in patients whose immune status is somewhere between that of patients with tuberculoid or lepromatous disease. Nerve damage is common and skin lesions vary in number and character. Neuropathic ulcers are a particular problem (**Fig. 15.42**).

DIAGNOSIS

Leprosy may be suspected clinically but the diagnosis needs to be confirmed by demonstrating acid-fast bacilli. This can be done by making skin smears from cool parts of the body (e.g. ear lobes, scapulae, buttocks) or histologically by skin biopsies (**Fig. 15.43**) or nerve biopsies.

TREATMENT

Successful management of leprosy relies on careful examination and documentation of nerve and skin lesions. Multidrug therapy is now standard for all types of leprosy and involves daily treatment with dapsone and clofazimine and monthly doses of rifampicin, plus a large dose of clofazimine for lepromatous disease. Treatment should continue for at least 2 years. Dapsone and rifampicin for at least 6 months is required for tuberculoid leprosy. Supervised monthly doses and good defaulter tracing are essential in endemic areas. In addition to chemotherapy, surgery may be required to correct deformity in chronic disease and to save sight when the eyes are involved.

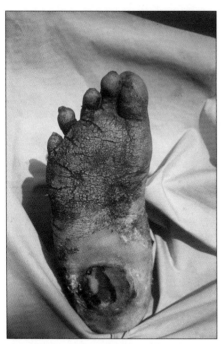

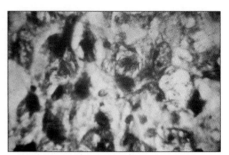

Fig. 15.43 *Skin biopsy showing numerous acid-fast bacilli (*Mycobacterium leprae*).*

Fig. 15.42 *Neuropathic foot ulcer in leprosy.*

LEPROSY REACTIONS

Type 1 lepra reactions

Sometimes during treatment, particularly in borderline leprosy, cell-mediated immunity may improve. The delayed hypersensitivity reaction that results may lead to swelling and erythema of skin lesions, peripheral oedema and painful swelling of nerves, sometimes with paralysis. These are called type 1 lepra reactions.

Type 2 lepra reactions

A second type of reaction, type 2 lepra reaction or erythema nodosum leprosum, is an immune complex phenomenon. Erythema nodosum leprosum may occur several months into treatment, but untreated patients may also present *de novo* with it. Systemic features, such as fever and myalgia, are common and erythema nodosum lesions appear on the extremities; these are often very tender. Nerve pain, epididymo-orchitis, bone pain and iritis may all occur.

Both types of leprosy reaction require analgesia and steroid therapy. Thalidomide is especially useful in erythema nodosum leprosum. Appropriate physiotherapy, including splinting, is required for neuritis.

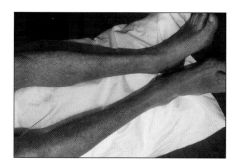

Fig. 15.44 *Skin rash in dengue fever.*

VIRAL INFECTIONS

DENGUE

There are four serotypes of dengue virus. All of these are spread by mosquitoes, usually *Aedes aegypti*. Dengue virus is widely distributed in the tropics. Usually, infection results in a self-limiting condition, dengue fever, sometimes known as breakbone fever. There is an abrupt onset of fever and rigors with severe backache, myalgia and arthralgia. As the fever wanes, an erythematous macular rash appears (**Fig. 15.44**) and there may be generalized lymphadenopathy. Sometimes, a second fever peak follows, the so-called 'saddleback fever.' Thrombocytopenia is common during the illness.

Occasionally, particularly in children in endemic areas, dengue haemorrhagic fever occurs as a complication. This is characterized by increased vascular permeability, shock and abnormal clotting. Dengue haemorrhagic fever is thought to result from a second infection with a different serotype in patients who are already immune to dengue after infection with another serotype of the virus, and immunological mechanisms are believed to lead to disease. It may occur in epidemics if a new serotype is introduced into a susceptible population.

YELLOW FEVER

Like dengue, yellow fever is caused by a mosquito-borne flavivirus. However, it is much more severe and is characterized by fever and rigors, followed a few days later by a progressive hepatitis and coagulopathy. Case fatality rates in epidemics may be as high as 40%. Also, unlike dengue, a good vaccine exists and can be used in epidemics to reduce the number of susceptible people.

VIRAL HAEMORRHAGIC FEVERS

In addition to the viral infections mentioned above, a variety of viruses may lead to severe febrile illnesses with shock and bleeding diatheses. Fortunately, these are rare and geographically limited. They are listed in **Figure 15.45**.

Viral haemorrhagic fevers

Disease	Virus type	Reservoir	Vector	Geographical distribution
Argentinian haemorrhagic fever	Arenavirus	Rodents	Tick	Pampas of Argentina
Bolivian haemorrhagic fever	Arenavirus	Rodents	Tick	Plains of Bolivia
Lassa fever	Arenavirus	Mice	None	Savannah of West Africa
Ebola virus disease	Filovirus	?	None	Savannah of eastern, central and southern Africa
Marburg virus disease	Filovirus	?	None	
Rift Valley fever	Phlebovirus	Mammals (wild and domestic)	Mosquito	Sub-Saharan Africa
Crimean–Congo haemorrhagic fever	Nairovirus	Various mammals	Tick	Africa, Asia, eastern Europe
Haemorrhagic fever with renal syndrome	Hantavirus	Mice, rats, voles	None	Asia, eastern Europe
Omsk haemorrhagic fever	Flavivirus	Musk-rats, voles	Tick	Eastern Europe
Kyasanur Forest haemorrhagic fever	Flavivirus	Monkeys	Tick	India
Yellow fever	Flavivirus	Monkeys	Mosquito	Tropical Africa and South America
Dengue fever	Flavivirus	Monkeys, humans	Mosquito	Widespread in tropics

Fig. 15.45 *Viral haemorrhagic fevers.*

MISCELLANEOUS TROPICAL CONDITIONS

TROPICAL ULCER

Tropical ulcer is an indolent condition caused by *Mycobacterium ulcerans*. Lesions usually affect the lower limbs and start as small nodules that subsequently become fluctuant and ulcerate (**Fig. 15.46**). Although most ulcers eventually heal, there may be significant oedema and local deformity as a result. The best treatment is surgical excision at an early stage. Chemotherapy has little role.

MYIASIS

Myiasis is infestation by larvae of flies. Larvae or maggots may contaminate wounds or sores. However, sometimes the larvae develop from eggs deposited on skin and burrow into normal skin. This creates a sort of furuncle, or boil, with a central sinus through which the larvae may sometimes be seen (**Figs 15.47** and **15.48**). Treatment requires removal of the larvae either by plugging the sinus with vaseline to promote larval exit or, more commonly, surgical removal by way of a cruciate incision.

MYCETOMA

In some areas of the tropics, various species of actinomyces or fungi may be implanted in the tissues of the foot after (often minor) penetrating injuries (**Fig. 15.49**). Locally destructive disease may lead to severe disability over time. Drugs have little impact on most of these infections and amputation is frequently required to relieve pain.

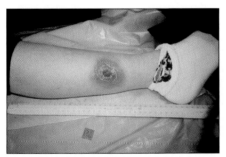

Fig. 15.46 *Tropical ulcer.*

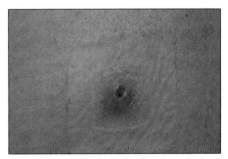

Fig. 15.47 *Typical skin lesion in myiasis.*

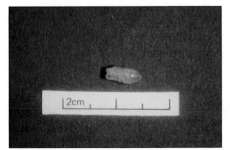

Fig. 15.48 *Excised fly larva from lesion in Fig. 15.47.*

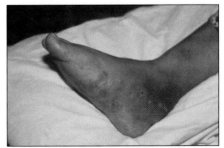

Fig. 15.49 *Mycetoma (madura foot) caused by* Pseudoallescheria boydii.

PYOMYOSITIS

This is a multifocal infection, usually staphylococcal, of skeletal muscle that occurs in the tropics, particulary in areas of high humidity. Affected muscles are usually painful and feel woody hard. Pink pus may be aspirated to clinch the diagnosis. Treatment requires a combination of antibiotics and surgical drainage.

AMOEBIC MENINGOENCEPHALITIS

Rarely, free-living amoebae (*Acanthamoeba* spp. and *Naegleria fowleri*) can invade the central nervous system and lead to either acute or chronic infections. The disease is most prevalent in southeast Asia. Diagnosis is difficult, as is treatment, and many cases end fatally.

TRAVEL MEDICINE

The availability of relatively cheap air travel means that millions of people can travel to the tropics and therefore run the risk of acquiring tropical diseases and, sometimes, returning home with them. The risks of acquiring these problems can be reduced by appropriate advice and immunizations before travel. The most important aspect of this is appropriate advice about preventing malaria. Details of malaria chemoprophylaxis are beyond the scope of this book. However, it is important to emphasize the reduction of mosquito bites by wearing appropriate clothing, using insect repellant and using mosquito nets at night. Drugs commonly used to prevent malaria include chloroquine, proguanil, mefloquine and doxycycline. Vaccinations that should be considered, depending on the trip planned, are highlighted in **Figure 15.50**. In addition, travellers should take a first-aid kit, sunscreen,

Vaccines for international travellers			
Vaccine	**Type**	**Route of administration**	**Re-immunization**
Polio (Salk)	Killed whole virus	i.m.	5–10 years
**Polio (Sabin)	Live attenuated virus	oral	5–10 years
Diphtheria	Adsorbed toxoid	i.m.	10 years
Tetanus	Adsorbed toxoid	i.m.	10 years
Yellow fever	Live attenuated virus	i.m.	10 years
**Typhoid (Vi)	Capsular polysaccharide	i.m.	3 years
Typhoid (Ty21a)	Live attenuated virus	oral	3 years
**†Hepatitis A vaccine	Killed whole virus	i.m.	10 years
***Meningococcal	Polysaccharide (types A&C)	i.m.	3 years
***Rabies	Killed whole virus	i.m. or i.d.	3–5 years
***Japanese B enceph.	Killed whole virus	i.m.	3 years
***Hepatitis B	Recombinant viral surface antigen	i.m. (i.d.)	5 years
***BCG	Live attenuated mycobacteria	i.d.	none

*Following full initial course of immunization
**Required for most travellers to the tropics
***Only required in certain circumstances
†Hepatitis A may also be prevented by administering i.m. human gammaglobulin which can confer protection for up to 4–6 months

Fig. 15.50 *Vaccines for travellers.*

Infective causes of fever in returning travellers	Infective causes of rash in returning travellers
Short incubation period (< 3 weeks) Malaria African trypanosomiasis Dengue fever Typhoid Tick typhus Hepatitis A Brucellosis Viral haemorrhagic fevers **Longer incubation period (> 3 weeks)** Malaria Brucellosis Liver abscess Typhoid Visceral leishmaniasis Hepatitis B, C or E Tuberculosis Primary HIV infection Filariasis	Cutaneous larva migrans Cutaneous leishmaniasis Dengue fever Tinea (dermatophyte infections) Lyme disease Infestations (lice, scabies) Tick typhus Typhoid (rose spots) Herpes simplex infection Sexually transmitted diseases (e.g. syphilis) Primary HIV infection

Fig. 15.52 *Infective causes of rash in returning travellers.*

Fig. 15.51 *Infective causes of fever in returning travellers.*

simple analgesics, antidiarrhoeal medication, oral rehydration sachets and any regular medication required.

RETURNING TRAVELLERS

Most travellers return unscathed from the tropics but some return with symptoms. Although many of these problems are self-limiting, others require specific treatment; again malaria is the most notable of these. Awareness of the possibility of imported disease is important for both patient and doctor. The two most frequent reasons why returning travellers seek medical advice are fever and skin rash. The most common causes of these symptoms are shown in **Figures 15.51** and **15.52**.

Index

Note: Page references in *italics* refer to Figures

A

abscess 130-1
  amoebic 116-17, *117*
  appendix 122
  Bartholin's 138, *138*
  brain 80-1, *80-1*
  cold 187
  corticomedullary *130*
  dental 54, *58*
  epidural 81-2
  hydatid cysts 117-18
  intra-abdominal 123, *123*
  intrathoracic 70
  liver 115-18
  lung 70-1, *71*
  pancreatic 120, *121*, *123*
  parapharyngeal 59, 60
  pelvic *178*
  perinephric 130-1, *131*
  periodontal 54
  peritonsillar 59, *59*
  perivalvular 43
  prostatic 135
  psoas 163, *164*
  pyogenic 115-16, *116*
  renal 40, 43, 130
  retropharyngeal 60, *60*
  splenic 40, *41*, 43, *43*
  tubulo-ovarian 152
  valve ring 39, 43
Acanthamoeba 92, 250
  A. castellani 92
  A. polyphaga 92
aciclovir 84, 91, 92, 95, 96, 168, 195, 212
Acinetobacter 156
adenovirus 91, *91*, 92
adherence, bacterial 2
adult respiratory distress syndrome 5, 6
Aedes aegypti 247
Aeromonas 226
African tick typhus 243
AIDS 35, 95, 171, 202
albendazole 233, 235, 236, 239
allopurinol 225
amikacin 94
aminoglycoside 62, 90, 119
amoebic dysentery 116
amoebic meningoencephalitis 250
amoxycillin 55, 140
amphotericin B 92, 198, 199, 225, 226
ampicillin 55
Ancylostoma braziliense 233
Ancylostoma duodenale 107, 231, 232

Anopheles 217
  A. gambiae 32
anorectal disease 138
anthrax 158, 159
antibiotics, classes and modes of action *4*
antibodies 3
anti-HBc 113
anti-HBsAg IgG 113
antimicrobial sensitivity testing 17-18
Antimicrobic Test System 17
aortic graft infection 50
aorto-duodenal fistula *50*
API test kit 17
arachidonic acid 6
arboviruses 84, *85*
artemisinine 221
Ascaris lumbricoides 107, *107*, 231, *232*
aspergilloma 72, 74
aspergillosis 22, 26, 74, 200-1, *200*
  allergic bronchopulmonary 71
  invasive 72
Aspergillus 45, 71-2, 80, 92, 192, 200, *201*
asthma 64
astrovirus 101
ataxia telangiectasia 194
athlete's foot 35, 166, *167*
atrial septal defects 37
azithromycin 139, 141, 206

B

B lymphocytes 3
Bacillus anthracis 158
bacillus Calmette-Guérin (BCG) vaccination 75
Bacillus cereus 93, 103
bacteraemia, primary 25-6
bacteriuria, asymptomatic 129
balanitis, circinate *153*
Bartholin's abscess 138, *138*
Bartonella 39
benzathine penicillin 146, 147
benzonidazole 223
benzylpenicillin 67, 157, 158
b-hemolytic streptococci 22
b-lactam agents 62, 122, 133
bile solubility test 16
bilharzia 241
BK virus 209
blackwater fever 219
blastomycosis 83
blepharitis 89, *89*
bone, anatomy 175, *175*
bone marrow transplantation 200-1

Bordetella parapertussis 64
Bordetella pertussis 64
Borrelia 242-3, *243*
Borrelia burgdorferi 83, 86, 88
botulinum 88
botulism 88
bovine spongiform encephalopathy 87
breakbone fever 247
Brevibacterium 156
bronchiectasis 65, *65*, 66
bronchiolitis, acute 64, *64*
bronchitis 64-5
  acute 64
  chronic 65
bronchopulmonary dysplasia 20
broth dilution techniques 17
brucellosis 83, *180*
Brudzinski's sign 77
Brugia malayi 227
Bruton's X-linked agammaglobulinemia 193
Burkholderia cepacia 191, *191*, 192
burns 24, 162, *162*, 190

C

Calabar swellings 230
calculus
  prostatic 133, *133*
  renal 127
Calymmatobacterium granulomatis 151
Campylobacter 13, *13*, 88, 104
  C. fetus 107
Candida 24, 45, 49, 92, 99, *99*, *100*, 141, 167, 184, 191-2, 194-5, 197-8, *198*
  C. albicans 38, 141, 165, *165*
candidaemia 93
candidial infections of skin 165
candidiasis 80, 99, 200
  chronic mucocutaneous 195, *195*
  disseminated *200*
  oesophageal *198*, *200*
carbol fuchsia 11
carbuncles 157, *157*
cardiac failure 39-40
cardiac syphilis 145
caries, dental 35, 53
carmine dye 25
catalase test 16
cataract 93
catheter-related infections 24, 129, *129*, 190-1
cefotaxime 55
ceftazidime 94

ceftriaxone 140, 147
cellular immunity 3
  defects in 194-5
cellulitis 157-8, *158*
  preseptal 98, *98*
central nervous system shunt
  infections 79-80
cephalosporins 19, 67, 119,
  121, 147
cestodes 236-40
Chagas' disease 46, 108, *109*
chalazion 89
chancroid 150-1
chickenpox 54, 168, *169*
  pneumonia 65, *66*, 67
Chlamydia 31, 39, 45, 122, 135
  C. pneumoniae 64
  C. psittaci 69
  C. trachomatis 14, 15, 90,
    135, 138, 140-1, 151, 152
  in neonates 215, *215*
chloramphenicol 55, 90, 244
chloroquine 220, 221, 250
cholangiocarcinoma 120
cholangitis 119-20
cholecystitis 118-19, *118*
cholera 32, 101-2, *102, 103*
  toxin 2
cholesteatoma 63
choroidoretinitis 94-5, *96*
chronic granulomatous disease
  (CGD) 3, 192, *193*
Chryops 230
cidofovir 95
ciprofloxacin 112, 135
clarithromycin 100, 206
classical pathway 3
clindamycin 142, 156, 157, 207
clinical history 1
clofazimine 246
Clonorchis (*Opisthorcis*)
  sinensis 32, 120
Clostridium botulinum 88
Clostridium difficile 110-11,
  111, 191
Clostridium parvum 103
Clostridium perfringens 11,
  105, *106*, 161, 190
clubbing, finger 40, *41*, 65
clue cells 142, *142*
coagulase test 16, *16*
Coccidioides 198
  C. immitis 199, *200*
coccidiodomycosis 34, 83, 199,
  200
cold sores 167
colonic carcinoma *123*
common variable
  immunodeficiency 193
complement system 3 3
  C3 3
  deficiencies 3
complement, abnormalities of
  194

condylomata acuminata 148,
  149, 171
condylomata lata 142, *143*
congenital rubella syndrome
  172, 212-13, *213*
conjunctivitis 90-1
  acute haemorrhagic 91
  bacterial 90, *90*
  chlamydial 90
  phlyctenular 73
  viral 91
continuous ambulatory
  peritoneal dialysis (CAPD)
  122, *122*
corneal infections 91-2
corticosteroids 7, 76, 86, 96
Corynebacterium 156
  C. diphtheriae 57, *58*
  C. ulcerans 57
co-trimoxazole 108, 151, 207
Coxiella burnetii 39, 41, 69,
  243
coxsackievirus 45, 54, *54*, 91,
  170
C-reactive protein (CRP) 178
Creutzfeldt-Jakob disease 86-7,
  86
  new variant 87
Crohn's disease 106, 108, 163
Cryptococcus 198
  C. neoformans 78, 135
cryptosporidiosis 207
culture methods 13-14
cutaneous larva migrans 233
cyclosporin 159
cystic fibrosis 65, *66*, 191
cysticercosis 83, *83*, 237
cystitis
  acute uncomplicated 126
  acute symptomatic 129
  complicated 127, 129
  diagnosis 127-8
    based on culture 127-8
    nonculture methods 128
  prophylaxis 129-30
  treatment 128-9
cytomegalovirus 15, 21, 31, 56,
  83, 88, 95, *95*, 99, 101, 194
  congenital 211
  HIV infection 205-6, *207*
  meningoencephalitis 206, *206*
  pneumonia 196, *197*, 201
  post-transplantation 195-6,
  196, 198
  retinitis 205

D
dapsone 159, 246
delta virus 114
dendritic ulcer 92, *92*
dengue 247, *247*
  dengue haemorrhagic fever
  247
dental caries 35, 53

dermatophyte infections of skin
  165
dexamethasone 94, 237
Di George syndrome 194
diabetes mellitus 62, 103, 130,
  158, 161, 162, 178
  diabetic coma 71, 72
  diabetic feet 182-3
diarrhoea
  antibiotic-associated 110-11
  inflammatory 104-6
  noninflammatory 101-3
diethylcarbamazepine 229, 230
a-difluoromethylornithine 222
diphtheria 57-8, *57-8*, 88
diphtheroids 182
dipstick, urine 128, *128*
discitis 180, *180*
disseminated intravascular
  coagulation 5, 7
Down's syndrome 34
doxycycline 112, 141, 147,
  250
dysentery *104, 105*

E
ear infections 61-4
echinococcosis 237-9
Echinococcus granulosus 117,
  237, *238*
Echinococcus multilocularis 118
echocardiography 41, *41*
echoviruses 45
ecthyma 157
ecthyma gangrenosum 192,
  192, 200
ectoparasites 149-50
ectopic pregnancy 152
eczema herpeticum 167, *168*
empyema 70, *70*, 71
  of gallbladder 119, *119*
endemic disease 35
endocarditis 4, 18, 37-44, 93
  antibiotic therapy 41-3, *42*
  bacterial 18
  clinical manifestations 39-40
  culture-negative 38-9
  diagnosis 41
  gonococcal 139
  in intravenous drug abusers 38
  native-valve 37-8, *37*
  pathology 39
  prophylaxis 43-4, *44*
  prosthetic valve 38
  surgery 43, *43*
  treatment 41-3
  tricuspid 40
endometritis 140
endophthalmitis, infectious 93-4,
  96
  candidal 93, *94*
  diagnosis 93
  endogenous 93
  postoperative 93

endophthalmitis, infectious (contd)
  following trauma 93
  treatment 94
endoscopic retrograde cholangiopancreatography (ERCP) 119, *119*, 120
endotoxin 2, 5
endotracheal tube, contamination by 24
endovascular infections 48
Entamoeba histolytica 106, 116, *116*, 117
enteric fever syndrome 106, 107, *107*
enteric infections 101-12
Enterobacter 19
Enterobius 232
Enterobius vermicularis 235
Enterococcus faecalis 38
Enterococcus faecium 38-9
Enterocytozoon bieneusi 208, 209
enterotoxin A 110
enteroviruses 45, 61, 46, 83
  skin infections 170
entropion 91
epidemics 35
epidemiology, definition 29
Epidermophyton 165
epididymitis 135, 140
epididymo-orchitis 136, *136*
epidural space infection 81-2
epiglottitis, acute 54-5
epsillometer test (E test) 18, *18*
Epstein-Barr virus 15, 55, *56*, 88, 95
erysipelas 157, *158*
erysipeloid 159, *159*
Erysipelothrix rhusiopathiae 159
erythema infectiosum 173
erythema nodosum 73, 152
erythrocyte sedimentation rate (ESR) 178
erythromycin 90, 141, 151
Escherichia coli 2, 10, *11*, 13, *14*, 15, 70, 103, 119, 121, 125, *126*, *127*, 130, 132
espundia 224, *225*
exanthem subitum 173
exotoxin 2, 5
eyelids, infections of 89

F
Fasciola hepatica 120
femoro-popliteal graft infection 50, *50*, 51
fever, in returning travellers *251*
fièvre boutonneuse 243
filarial infections 227-9
filariasis 227-9, *228*
  bancroftian 227
  brugian 227
  lymphatic 227

Fitz-Hugh–Curtis syndrome 138
floppy baby syndrome 88
flucloxacillin 156
fluconazole 165, *195*, 198
flucytosine 92
flukes *242*
fluorescent stains 11-12
fluorescent treponemal antibody absorption test (FTA-Abs) 146
fluoroquinolones 90, 133, 183
folliculitis 157, *157*
foscarnet 95
Fourniere's gangrene 161, *161*
fungal skin infections 165-7
furuncles 157
Fusarium 92

G
gallbladder infections 118-20
gallstones 118, *118*, *119*
gammaglobulin 34
g-interferon 193
ganciclovir 95, 197
gangrene 7
  Fourniere's 161, *161*
  gas 32, 161-2, *190*
Gardnerella vaginalis 142
gastroenteritis 101
gastrointestinal tract, infections of 99-101
genital warts 148, *149*
giant cell granulomas 115, *115*
Giardia lamblia 103, *103*, 194, *194*
giardiasis 103, 217
gibbus 186
Giemsa stain 12
gingivitis 53, *53*
  acute necrotizing 53
  suppurative 53
glandular fever 55-6, *56*
glaucoma 93
Glossina 221
glycopeptides 67
Gomori stain 12
gonococcal infection 31, 138-9
  gonococcal ophthalmia neonatorum 215
gonorrhoea 35, 137-40
  diagnosis 139
  treatment 139-40
graft-versus-host disease 201, *201*
Gram-negative organisms 9, *9*, 24,25
Gram-positive organisms 9, *9*
Gram stain 9-11, *11*
granulocytopenia 26, 192
granuloma
  giant cell 115, *115*
  hepatic 115, *116*
  macular chorioretinal 96
  necrotizing 207
granuloma inguinale 151, *151*

granulomatous hepatitis 115
griseofulvin 166, 167
Guillain-Barré syndrome 88, 204

H
HACEK organisms 38, *39*, 41
haemolysis of red blood cells 190, *190*
haemolytic-uremic syndrome 15
Haemophilus 93
Haemophilus aegypticus 90
Haemophilus ducreyi 150
Haemophilus influenzae 10, *11*, 13, *13*, 62, 65, 78, *78*, 90, 98, 176-7, *194*
  type b 34, 54, *55*, 79
  vaccine 78
halofantrine 221
hand washing, effect of 27, *27*
Hansen's disease *see* leprosy
Hantavirus 32
HBV e antigen (HBeAg 113
HBV surface antigen (HBsAg) 113
head and neck space infections 58-60
Heaf test 75
heart murmurs 39
Helicobacter pylori 99-100, *100*
helminth infections 226-7
hepatic granuloma 115, *116*
hepatitis 112-15
hepatitis A virus 22, 25, 112-13, *112*
  immunization 34
hepatitis B virus 22, 113, *113*, *114*, 197
  carrier state 34
  incubation period 29
  needle-stick transmission 26
  transmission 31
hepatitis C virus 14, 22, 114, *115*, 197
  needle-stick transmission 26
  transmission 31
hepatitis E virus 114
hepatitis F virus 114
hepatitis G virus 114-15
hepatobiliary system
  infections of 112-20
  parasitic diseases 120
herpes simplex virus (HSV) 99, 147-8, *147*
  cellulitis 98
  conjunctivitis 91
  encephalitis 84, *84*
  in HIV 208
  keratitis 92, *92*
  meningitis 83
  mouth ulcers 54, *54*
  organ transplantation 195
  in pregnancy 212
  of skin 167-8, *168*
  type 1 94
  type 2 95

herpesvirus 94, 115, *115*, 211-12
  skin infections 167-8
herpes zoster 168
highly active antiretroviral
  therapy (HAART) 204
Hirschsprung's disease 108
Histoplasma 198, 200
  H. capsulatum 32, *33*, 46,
    106, 199, *199*
histoplasmosis 83, 199
hookworm 231-3
hordeolum (sty) 89, *89*
hospital, transmission in 21-6,
  21, 22
  commonly acquired infections
    23
  control 26-7
  site of infection 23
  sterilization and disinfection
    26-7
host defences 2-4
host susceptibility 34
human immunodeficiency virus
  (HIV) 14, *15*, 15, 22, 56, 61,
    83, 202-10, *202*
  abscess 135
  CMV infection 205-6, *206*
  congenital 213
  latent viruses 208-9
  molluscum contagiosum 170
  mycobacterial infections 206-7
  needle-stick transmission 26
  in oesophagus 99
  parasitic infections 207-8
  pathogens in *205*
  Pneumocystis carinii infection
    204-5, *206*
  pneumonia 67
  progressive multifocal
    leucoencephalopathy 87
  strongyloidiasis 233-5
  transmission 31
  transverse myelitis 88
human papillomavirus (HPV)
  148, 171
human T-lymphotropic virus
  type I 88
humoral immunity 3
hydatid cysts 117, *117*, 118
hypogammaglobulinaemia 67
hypoglobulinaemia *193*
hypoglycorrhachia 77
hypopyon 91, *91*, 92, 93

I
iatrogenic infections 19
  agents 19-21
imidazoles 92
immunization 34, *35*
  active 34
  passive 34
immunoblots 15
immunodeficiency 189, *189*
immunofluorescence 12, *15*

immunoglobulins (Ig) 3
  deficiency 193, 194
  IgG 15, 193-4
  IgM 15
impetigo 1, 156, *156*
incubation period 29-30, *30*
infectious mononucleosis 55
influenza 21, 22, 25, 61, 67
interferon-gamma 3, 6
interleukins
  IL-1 6
  IL-2 3
  IL-4 3
  IL-10 3
intertrigo *165*
intravenous drug usage 162-3,
  163
intravenous therapy,
  contamination by 24
ischaemic legs 158
isoniazid 76
Isospora belli 103, 208, *209*
itraconazole 165, 166, 167
ivermectin 230
Ixodes dammini 32, *32*

J
Janeway's lesions 40
Jarisch-Herxheimer reaction 243
JC virus 87, 209

K
Katayama fever 241
Kawasaki disease 173-4, *174*
keratitis
  amoebic 92
  bacterial 91-2
  fungal 92
  viral 92
keratoconjunctivitis 91
Kerning's sign 77
ketoconazole 195, 225
Kirby-Bauer sensitivity test 18,
  18
Klebsiella 119, 125, 130
Koplik spots 171, *172*
kuru 87

L
lactobacilli 53
Legionella 13, *13*, 45
Legionella pneumophila 15, 68
Legionnaires' disease 68, 69
Leishmania 223, 224
  L. aethiopica 224
  L. braziliensis 224, 225
  L. mexicana 224
  L. tropica 224
leishmaniasis 223-6
  American mucocutaneous
    224, *225*
  cutaneous 224-5, *225*
  leishmaniasis recidivans 224
  visceral 225-6, *226*

leishmanin test 225
leprosy 88, 244-6
  borderline 245
  lepromatous 245, *245*
  neuropathic foot ulcers in
    245, *245*
  tuberculoid 244-5, *245*
  type 1 lepra reactions 246
  type 2 lepra reactions 246
leucocoria 96
leucocyte 3
leukaemia 26
  acute myeloid 73
leukotrienes 6
ligase chain reaction 14
lipopolysaccharide 2, 5
Listeria monocytogenes 78, 79,
  215
  in pregnancy 215
listeriosis, neonatal 215
Loa loa 227, 230, *230*
Loeffler's syndrome 231, 232,
  233
Lowenstein-Jensen medium 74
Ludwig's angina 58, *59*
Lyme disease 31, 32, 45, 83, 86
lymphoedema 158
lymphogranuloma venereum
  151-2, *152*
lymphoma 26
lysozyme 3

M
MacConkey plate *14*
macrolides 69, 141
macrophages 3
major histocompatibility
  complex (MHC) 3
malaria 12, 32, 217-21
  algid 219
  benign tertian 220
  cerebral 219
  chemoprophylaxis 250
  clinical features 219-20
  control and prevention 221
  diagnosis 220
  falciparum 219, *219*
  patterns *33*
  resistance 32, *33*
  treatment 220-1
  vivax 220, *220*
Mantoux test 75, *76*
masticator space infection 58
mastoiditis 62, *63*
Mazotti test 229
measles (rubeola) 15, 21, 29,
  67, 87, 88, 171-2
  pneumonia 65
mebendazole 231, 233, 236
mefloquine 221, 250
melarsoprol 222
meningitis 4
  aseptic 82-3
  bacterial 18, 77-9, *78*, 80